DIY Beauty Collection:
150 Organic Homemade Skin Care Recipes

Table of content

The Complete Reference Guide of Essential Oils

Introduction

If you have spent any amount of time online, you know that it is important to watch what you are putting in or on your body. You know that there are medications and supplements that are meant to help your health in a variety of ways, but then you read that you should avoid a whole list of items that are then found in the supplements you are using.

So what do you do?

You know that you want to do the best thing for your health and your body, but what are you supposed to do when the very things you are supposed to use for your health end up being full of the very things you try to avoid.

You think of how you want to do what is best for your health, for your family, and for the planet, but you don't think you can do this if you are supporting the synthetic products that are on the shelves today.

This is a common feeling that a lot of people share, and thankfully the number one solution to this problem is also the solution to your health concerns. Essential oils are entirely natural, free of harmful synthetic chemicals, and can be used in more ways than any synthetic medication you could imagine.

You have a headache, you want to relax, and you want to settle the house down at the end of the day.

You don't want to turn to the synthetic medications that are full of warnings and things to watch for, but what do you do?

Essential oils is the answer. You can diffuse a few drops in a diffuser, you can apply a few drops directly to your skin, or you can even add certain kinds to tea, and you get the same great results.

Calm, quiet tranquility fills your home, and you feel better.

That's just the beginning. The more familiar you get with essential oils, the more you will be able to treat the ailments that arise, and the more natural you can live.

So are you ready to jump into the world of essential oils?

Naturally.

Chapter 1 – Getting Started

There is a lot of excitement when you start out in this journey, but before you just dive in and spread oils on everything, I want to get you started on the right track. This means you need to know what you are doing from the beginning.

You can't just toss essential oils around and see what happens, you have to know what each oil does, and how to use them for your particular symptoms. This is something you can use both ways. You can use this knowledge to use the right oil for your particular ailment, and you can avoid the oils that won't help you or potentially make you feel worse.

On the other hand, if you know what oils create different results, you will be able to set up your home with a lot of preventative aspects, meaning you won't get sick as often or feel the stress to begin with.

So, let's dive in and learn the facts about essential oils, how to use them, and what oils work well with each other.

Knowledge is an effective weapon.

The Wonder Oils

While each section you find is going to have its own list of oils, there are a few oils that seem to stand out from the rest. Yes, there are going to be times when you need to treat something specific, and you will need an equally specific oil to get the job done, but on the other hand, you are going to see a few oils show up time and time again, no matter what the ailment happens to be.

These are the oils I would like to refer to as the Wonder Oils, because there are so many ways using these oils can make your life better.

They are good for the specifics, and they are good for the broad categories.

Whether you are dealing with aches, pains, illness, insomnia, or want to promote things such as peace, tranquility, focus, happiness, and better relationships, these are the oils you always want to have on hand.

Peppermint

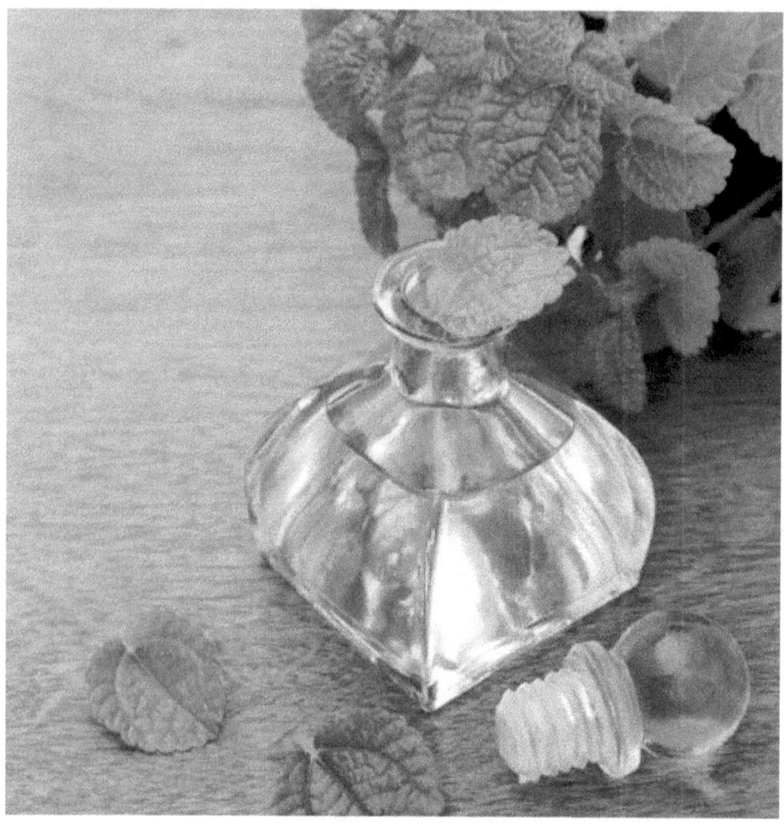

https://www.google.com/search?
q=peppermint+essential+oil&espv=2&biw=1366&bih=623&source=lnms&tbm=isch&sa=X&ved=0ahUKEwittoLvqo
LNAhVDM1IKHfg9BSMQ_AUIBygC#imgrc=ahsC9-zCsT80EM%3A

While many of us may associate this scent and taste with the holidays, there are a few things you need to know about this delightful oil that has nothing to do with Christmas trees or Santa Clause.

Peppermint oil has a light, fresh scent that blends exceptionally well with most other oils. It can be diffused for aroma therapy, applied topically on various aches and pains, and it can be enjoyed internally if it is highly diluted in water or tea. This oil is going to ease pains, clear your mind, and make you feel better and at peace.

It is abundantly available… you can purchase it not only online but in a variety of health and wellness stores to even large chain department stores. This oil truly is a wonder worker, and I suggest you keep plenty of it on hand at all times.

Lavender

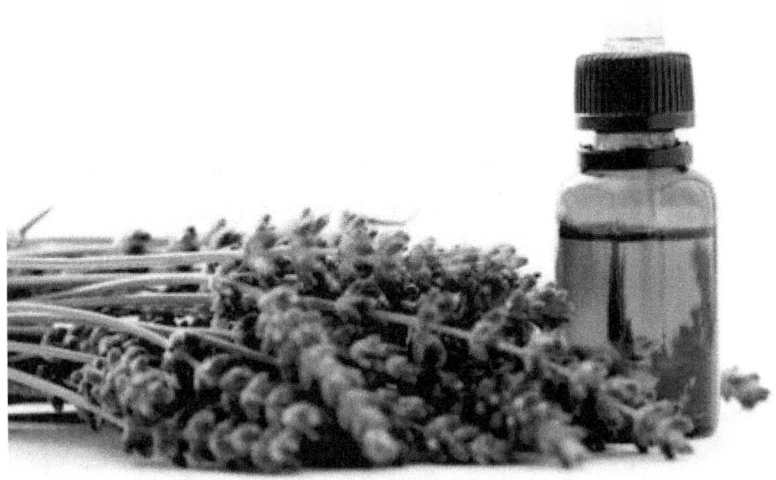

The floral scent of lavender is soothing to the mind, body, and soul. You would be amazed at how many people there are who think they don't like floral scents, but gravitate toward lavender.

Certainly among the best of the best, lavender is easily considered a Wonder Oil.

This oil is like peppermint in regards to the fact it will ease many of your life's ailments. Whether you are tense, stressed, or unable to sleep, a few drops of this oil spread across your forehead, blended into your bath water, or diffused in your bedroom is going to ease all of that tension that has built up and help you not only fall asleep, but stay asleep.

When you realize you can't become dependent on it, but you can use it as freely as you like, you are going to realize even more why you should keep this on hand at all times.

Make a space in your cabinet to house your lavender, peppermint, and tea tree oils, and there are few things you will face that you won't be able to handle.

Tea tree

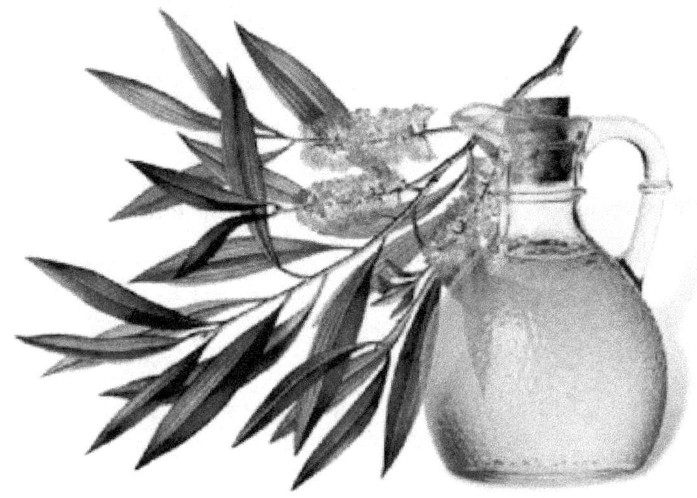

When it comes to physical ailments and imperfections, few things are going to do more for you than tea tree oil. While this oil has a strong, somewhat overwhelming scent, the benefits it does for your skin are far beyond the strong scent it holds.

Tea tree oil is a natural antiseptic. You can apply it to scrapes, cuts, and even acne and it will heal and clear up the imperfection. Excellent for hair, skin, and even sore throats and coughs, this oil is best diffused into the air for aroma therapy or mixed with a carrier oil and applied topically.

If you want to lighten the scent of this Wonder Oil, you can blend it with less offensive oils such as lavender, rose, or lemon. Another terrific benefit that comes with tea tree oil is that it is even more abundant than peppermint or lavender. You can purchase large vials of the purest form online or in health food stores, and it doesn't cost nearly as much as some of the more exotic oils do.

This oil's benefits far outweigh the scent, so make sure to get a large vial of it and keep it up in your cabinet along with the lavender and peppermint. You will be so glad you did.

Chapter 2 – The Best of the Blends

You may only be experiencing one feeling, or you may want to promote a singular feeling, in which case you only need to choose the oil or oils that you enjoy. There are going to be times, however, when you need to address more than one problem at a time, or when you want to create a blend of energy in your home.

To do this, you need to combine oils in properly to get the desired effect.

Thankfully, blending oils is not only easy, it is encouraged to create the best fragrances and optimum results, so you won't have any problem at all finding the right blend for your needs.

The trick to getting the best of the blends is to know how to blend the oils yourself

If you get online, you are going to find that there are plenty of blends all ready to go. The supplier puts them together and sells them as a blend, usually under the name of what you need it for.

For example, you can purchase an oil blend from Doterra called "On Guard". It is an immunity support oil, but if you look closer at it, you will see that it is, in fact, a blend of the everyday oils you have on hand such as wild orange, clove bud, cinnamon, eucalyptus, and rosemary.

While there is a lot of convenience to purchasing the oil already blended, you are going to find that you will save a lot of money, and get a lot more of the product if you purchase the oils separately and blend them yourself.

Wait, purchasing all of those oils separately isn't going to be inexpensive... the blend is a lot cheaper to buy as it is

Yes, that may be true, but if you think about it, if you purchase the ingredients separately, not only do you get enough to make the blend yourself, but you also get the extra oils left over to put to other use.

This is going to come in handy if you want to have the immunity support, as well as treat any ailment you already have, or simply to set some aside until you need it again. You see, when you are blending the oils yourself, you always have a lot of each on hand, simply because you only use a few drops of each one when you do use it.

So that brings us to the actual blending aspect.

When you blend the oils yourself, make sure you look at the total number of drops you are going to be using at the end result. If you are making enough to save some, keep the ratios the same, but if you are only mixing one time use at a time, watch out for how much you are actually using.

What this means is that if you are going to use the oils to make the equivalent to Doterra's On Guard, you need to realize that the 2 drops you use from that bottle are 2 blended drops.

I know that sounds confusing at first, but think about it this way. If you are mixing in the On Guard into your tea to sip on, you only need 1 or 2 drops to do it. All of those oils I listed that create this blend come together in those 2 drops you put into your tea.

If you were to take each of those drops and place only 1 drop each in your tea separately, then you will end up with 5 or 6 drops, which is simply too much to ingest at one time. If you put this all in your tea at once, you will run into problems from overdosing on the oils.

To get around this, you need to cut back on the amount of oils you are using in your tea, or (better yet) blend them all separately then take 2 drops of what you have blended. The most important thing you need to remember when it comes to essential oils is that you can overdose, and too much of some of them can be toxic.

Keep small jar glasses on hand, or purchase some of your own vials to store the extra oils you blend. This is going to keep them safe until you need them again, and help you stay on track with the proper dosage of the oils.

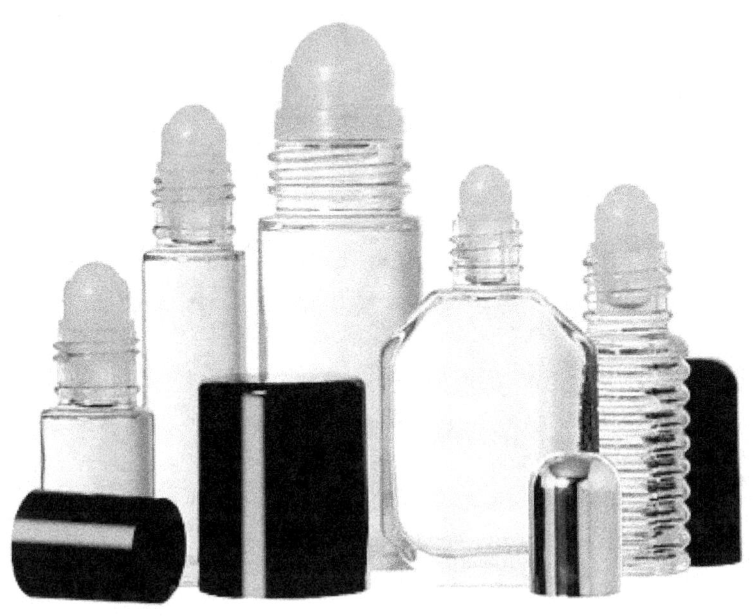

Small vials that have the drop lid are available online, or you can even get them locally at a number of stores. One of the major benefits to mixing your own blends in your own bottles is that you get to then choose the bottles you want to use as well.

This means you can create your own mists, roll ons, or drop bottles to suit your own taste, and keep them on hand where you want them. Say you want to take an anti-stress blend to work with you? No problem!

Purchase a roll on dispenser, mix up your favorite blend or just use your favorite anti-stress oil, fill your roll on dispense, and toss it in your purse. No matter where your day goes you will have your instant anti-stress mechanism at just an arm's length away, and your day is going to go so much better.

When you are creating your own blends, start with the desired effect you want your blend to have, and move on from there.

For example, if you want a blend that is going to help you sleep, but you also want to relieve tension and stress besides, start with the lavender. You want there to be more lavender in this blend than anything else, so I would recommend starting with 10 or 12 drops of this oil.

Then, pick the other oils you want. Peppermint is great for stress relief, so choose this one next, but don't put in the same amount. Perhaps 6 or 7 drops to suit your own taste.

What you want to keep in mind is that you want to use the most of your main focus, then add in the secondary oils as secondary benefits. Once you have this down, you can make any blend you want for any use you want.

Get creative!

Chapter 3 – Oils by Symptoms or Desired Effect

There are times when you are looking through the oils to see what they do, but there are also times when you feel a certain way and you want to find the oils that make it better.

What I mean by this is that you may enjoy the smell of rose oil and lavender oil, so you diffuse this in your home often. You are going to gain the amazing benefits that come from diffusing this oil… which means you are going to feel calm, relaxed, open, etc… but this doesn't help when you are suffering from a headache.

So, if you happen to have some sort of ailment (a headache, a stomach ache, a tooth ache), you need to know which oils to use specifically for these problems.

Here are oils separated into categories based on the symptoms you feel.

You can use one of the oils in the category, or you can mix and match as you please to take care of many of your symptoms.

Body Aches and Pains

Body aches and pains are annoying as well as debilitating. When you feel any of these symptoms, you know you want to get better as soon as possible.

I suggest for any of the oils or oil blends you use here, mix a few drops with a carrier oil and massage onto the aching area.

You can also add 10 to 12 drops into a warm bath and soak your pain away.

Headaches

Eucalyptus

Lavender

Peppermint

Stomach aches

Peppermint

Ginger

Roman chamomile

Melissa

Star anise

Grapefruit

Spearmint

Cardamom

Coriander

Fennel

Aniseed

Joint pain and stiffness

Sweet marjoram

Chamomile

Rosemary

Peppermint

Eucalyptus

Muscle cramps

Peppermint

Lemongrass

Basil

Vetiver

Sage

Cypress

Grapefruit

Rosemary

Natural Cold and Flu Remedies

When it comes to treating the cold and flu, I suggest you use a diffuser next to your bed or couch. The oils will fill the air and the aroma therapy will clear the illness right out.

If you are dealing with specific aches such as a sore throat, cough, or headache, you may also mix the oils of your choice with a carrier oil and massage it into the infected area, or add a drop or two to tea and sip on it.

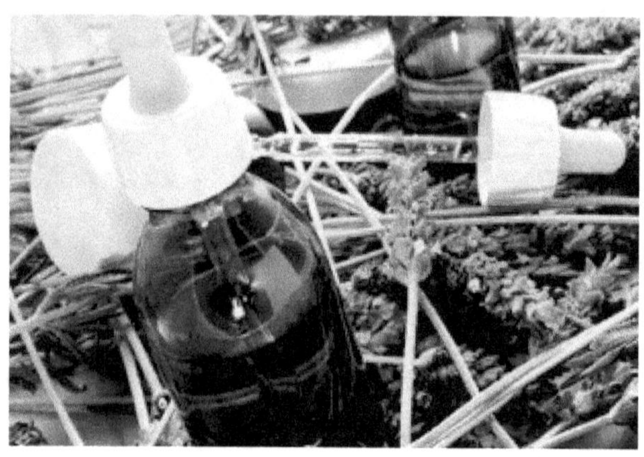

https://www.google.com/search?
q=essential+oil+skin+care&espv=2&biw=1366&bih=623&site=webhp&source=lnms&tbm=isch&sa=X&ved=0ahUK
Ewj2qvG1qYLNAhUNSFIKHSunCKIQ_AUIBygC#imgrc=Bh2o8B1JeDrWnM%3A

Colds

Lavender

Eucalyptus

Thyme

Rosemary

Garlic

Sandalwood

Lemon

Chamomile

Peppermint

Sore Throat

Eucalyptus

Oregano

Sage

Tea tree

Ginger

Peppermint

Cough

Lavender

Peppermint

Lemongrass

Frankincense

Lemon

Stress

No matter what kind of job you work or what kind of life you live, you are going to deal with a level of stress.

To rid your mind and body of that stress, I strongly suggest you use these oils or any blend of these oils in a diffuser, or add 10 to 12 drops into your hot bath water before you soak in the tub.

Tension

Helichrysum

Peppermint

Spearmint

Roman chamomile

Eucalyptus

Lavender

Insomnia

Lavender

Roman chamomile

Sweet marjoram

Vetiver

Ylang ylang

Anxiety

Basil

Clary sage

Bergamot

Frankincense

Ylang ylang

Marjoram

Peppermint

The Air of the House is the Mood of the Home

They say prevention is the best cure, and if you set up your home to be a safe haven, you are going to skip out on a lot of stressful symptoms that pop up in day to day life.

Use these oils in diffusers around your home. Diffusers aren't expensive and they are easy to maintain.

Prevent ailments and issues and promote peace and health with these oils blended into the air of your home at all times.

The Essentials you will need:

To promote tranquility

Chamomile

Roman chamomile

Lavender

Cedar wood

To promote happiness

Orange

Rose

Jasmine

Ginger

Cloves

Sandalwood

Petitgrain

Frankincense

Lemon

Geranium

To promote energy

Black pepper

Bergamot

Grapefruit

Peppermint

Rosemary

Thyme

Lemon

Basil

Fennel

To promote peace

Tangerine

Orange

Patchouli

Ylang ylang

Cassia

Davana

German chamomile

Cistus

Lavender

Lemon

Chapter 4 – The Practical Side of Things

In life there are far more things we want to address and take care of besides mood and colds. You want beautiful hair, you want to lose weight or maintain a weight loss. Your teenagers want clear skin and you want to avoid or get rid of the wrinkles that somehow appeared around your mouth and eyes.

Sure, it's great to know how to address a headache or sleeplessness, but once you know how to also get rid of such things as acne, wrinkles, and oily hair, you are going to be completely taken care of in your oil usage.

That is why I have included this chapter, so you know exactly what you can use to treat or prevent those physical imperfections you don't want to have to deal with any longer.

And when you combine the fact you get to save money as well as save your skin from harmful chemicals, you have a complete win, and everyone wants to have that.

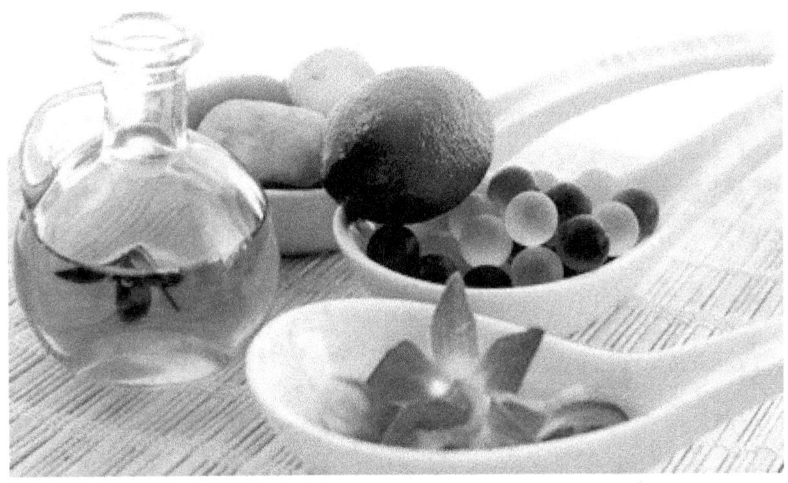

https://www.google.com/search?q=essential+oil+skin+care&espv=2&biw=1366&bih=623&site=webhp&source=lnms&tbm=isch&sa=X&ved=0ahUKEwj2qvG1qYLNAhUNSFIKHSunCKIQ_AUIBygC#imgrc=Bh2o8B1JeDrWnM%3A

People of all ages across the globe spend hundreds and thousands of dollars each year on various skin care products. Each of the products claim they are going to do the magic trick, but most of them end up not working anyway.

Not to mention these products are full of chemicals you don't want on your skin. Using essential oils are always a better choice, and I promise you that you are going to see better results using these than you ever did with store products.

To use these, mix with your face soap, moisturizer, or with a carrier oil and apply directly to the spot you want to focus on.

How to get rid of acne

Jojoba

Lavender

Tea tree

Orange

Frankincense

Get rid of those wrinkles!

Myrrh

Frankincense

Rose

Carrot seed

Lavender

Geranium

Sandalwood

Minimize the appearance of pores and say goodbye to freckles

Lemon

Tea tree

Lemongrass

Carrot seed

Geranium

Frankincense

Many commercials proudly proclaim that your hair is as unique as you, but you don't find this to be a good thing when you can't find any product that does what you need it to do.

Here are the oils you want to turn to based on what you need for your hair. Blend a few drops in with your shampoo and wash as you normally would.

The results are real, and you are going to love them.

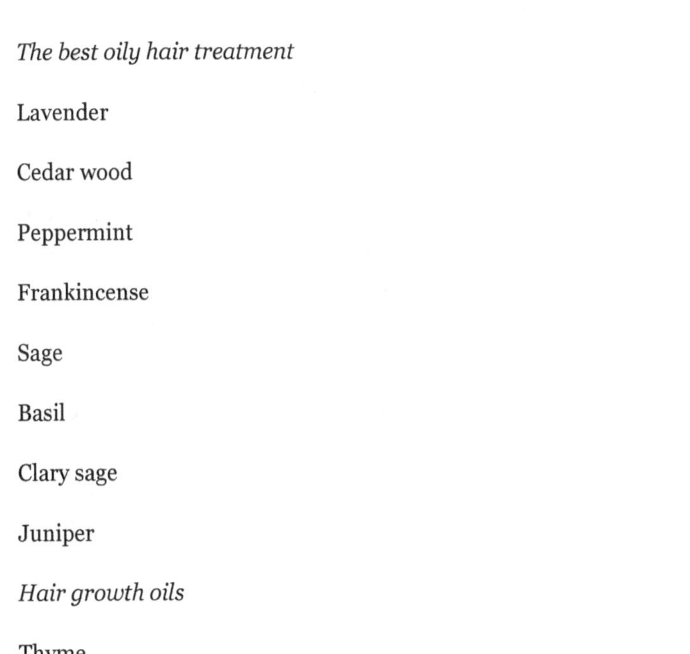

The best oily hair treatment

Lavender

Cedar wood

Peppermint

Frankincense

Sage

Basil

Clary sage

Juniper

Hair growth oils

Thyme

Lavender

Rosemary

Moisture for the dry hair

Clary sage

Lemon

Thyme

Tea tree

Cedar wood

Weight Loss and Weight Management

It seems that majority of people want to lose weight, but once they do, it is a struggle to keep it off. If you bring in these oils, you are going to see the weight melt away, as well as keep it off for good.

I suggest you use a diffuser for these oils, or that you highly dilute a drop or two into a tall glass of water. The results are real, entirely natural, and not even remotely dangerous.

You really can lose that weight for good, and enjoy the results, knowing they are going to last.

Essential weight loss

Lemon

Grapefruit

Cypress

Ginger

Peppermint

Cinnamon

Garlic

Perfect weight management

Grapefruit

Tangerine

Lemon

Spearmint

Ocotea

Cinnamon bark

Thieves

And, of course…. Peppermint

I'm sure you saw the overlap I mentioned in chapter 1 of all the ways you can use the top 3 oils, but I do strongly urge you to go out and get as many oils as you can find. They have dozens for sale on Amazon, or you can look into the other private suppliers that are around both online and locally.

No matter where you decide to get your essential oils, the important thing you need to remember is to check that they are pure. A pure essential oil is going to come in a dark bottle, as this is the best way to store them. The liquid itself is going to be strongly scented, and have an oily appearance just by looking at it.

If you get your oils from reputable sources, you have nothing to worry about, so just go through somewhere you trust, and make sure it says on the label that it is 100% pure before you buy.

Chapter 5 – The Tricks of the Trade: How to Use Essential Oils

You can know all kinds of things about essential oils, whether it be which ones are best for certain symptoms, what blends smell the best, or what kind of oils you want to avoid in various situations, but all of this is just head knowledge unless you know how to take them from the vial and put them into your life.

There are a number of different methods that people use when it comes to essential oils.

The most common are:

1. Diffusing

2. Applying topical

3. Taking internally

Let's take a moment now to look at each one, and you can decide which method you prefer for yourself, or what combination of methods you want to use. Some people choose one, others combine one or two, then there are those that use all three, the great thing about essential oils and knowing how to use them is that you can do what you want, when you want it.

Diffusing

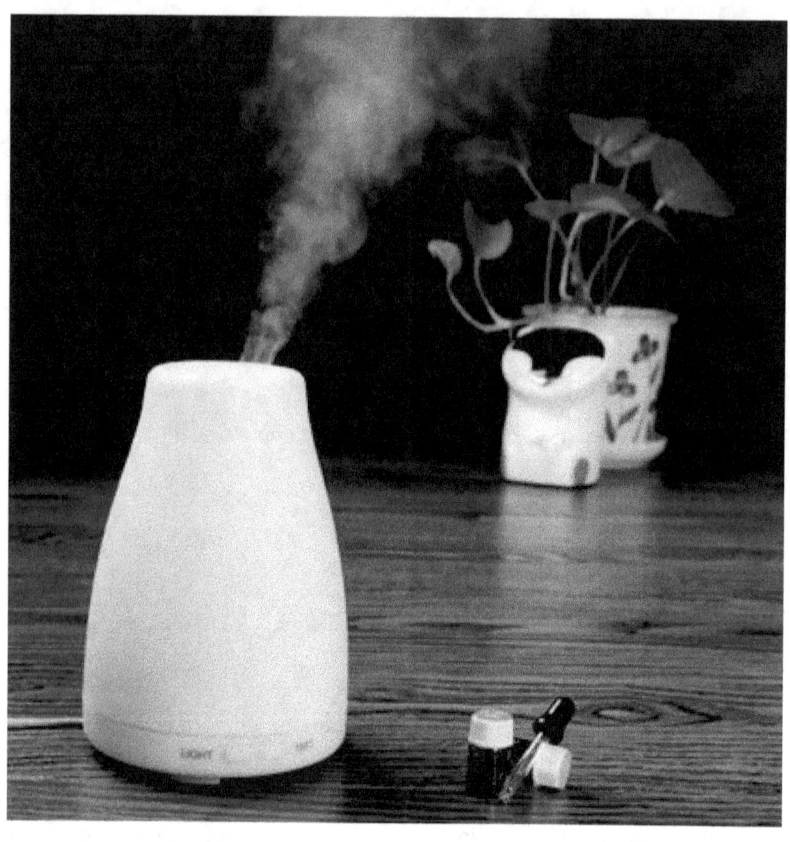

The most common method of using essential oils is diffusing. To do this, you purchase a diffuser, fill it with water (the amount of water varies with the diffuser you purchase), and add a few drops of oil.

If you know the specific symptom you want to treat, you put in the oil or blend of oils into the diffuser, plug it in, and let it fill the air with a delightful smelling mist. The aroma therapy treats the ailment, and makes your house smell incredible.

Topical use

Another prevalent method is applying the oil topically. When you do this, you still choose the oil you want based on the symptoms that are at hand. For example, you know that peppermint helps with stomach aches and lavender helps with restlessness, so if you are dealing with the stomach flu, a blend of these two oils will help a lot.

To apply topically, you are only going to use a few drops total, perhaps 2 drops of each oil.

Now, many oils are harsh applied directly to your skin, so you need to be careful with the oils you are using. The best way to prevent any skin irritation is to combine the oil with a carrier oil.

Carrier oils are mild oils that can be applied liberally to any part of your body, they are usually common oils such as coconut, sunflower, olive oil, or even vegetable oil if you are in a pinch.

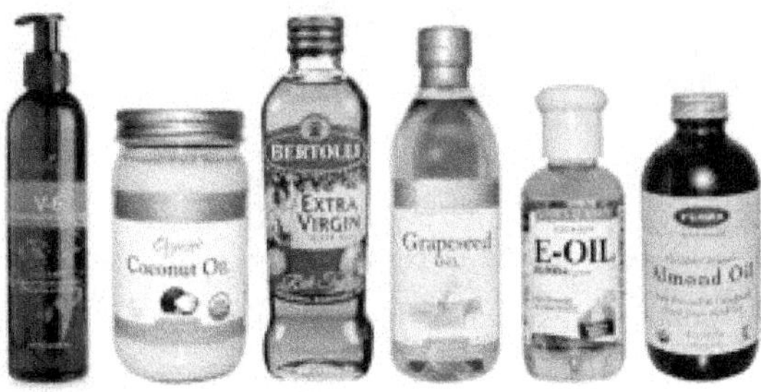

The best ratio I have found with the essential oil and the carrier oil is to combine a few drops of the essential oil with half a tablespoon of the carrier oil. Spread this on the part that is ailing (massage it into your forehead, onto your stomach, or any joint that is ailing. I find that it helps to warm the oil slightly before massaging it into your body.

Taking the Oil Internally

There is a lot of debate when it comes to ingesting essential oils. Many people advise against it because there can be harmful side effects, or you can overdose on the oils if you don't follow the dosages.

In my experience, I have never had an issue taking a couple drops of oil in my tea, but I am always careful of proper dosages. If you are going to use it in your tea, only use a couple of drops, no matter how big your cup of tea is. Only do this once a day.

Sure, there is the tendency to think that if 2 drops is good, then 4 must be better, but that is not the case. Essential oils are highly concentrated, which means the couple drops you are using in your tea is the equivalent to a lot of the fruit or other substance you are using.

Go mild, blend it into the tea you are drinking, and remember that less is more. If you feel sick, dizzy, or like something is off, discontinue ingesting the oils and simply use them topically or diffused into the air. There is evidence to support that you get the same benefits from using these oils topically or through aroma therapy as there is ingesting it.

At the end of the day, you get to decide what you want to do. It's your body, you get to decide. Don't be afraid to try out all three and decide which you want to do for yourself, and have fun with it!

My goal with this book is to give you the freedom you deserve to have with your health, and using essential oils is the best way to do that.

Conclusion

There you have it, everything you need to know to get well versed in the use of essential oils. With this book, you will know not only what kind of oils to use for certain ailments, but you will also know which blends to make and how to administer for the greatest results.

Discover your perfect method, combine that with your favorite blends, and reap the excellent benefits that are sure to follow. In no time at all you will know just what to do with any ailment that arises, no matter what time of the day it is.

I hope this book is able to show you how you can treat any ailment naturally, and you can do it your way. No strict rules, no crazy side effects to worry about, and absolutely none of that medicinal smell that you don't want on you or your children.

Natural remedies are by far the best way to go, and when you know what you are doing, you have the very key you need to make it happen. That is what this book aims to do, and that is exactly what you will be able by the time you have reached this point.

I hope you now feel the confidence I know you should have, and that you are able to treat and prevent a variety of ailments that arise in day to day living. These treatments are the best of the best. They have been around for thousands of years for a reason… they work!

Forget the stress that comes from going to the store and standing in the medication aisle for hours, trying to decide which one is best for you. Now, you can treat anything you can think of naturally, and naturally you can do it whenever you please.

Essential Oil Recipes for Diffusers

Introduction

It is really enjoyable to use essential oil blends in a diffuser and enjoy the benefits of aromatherapy. You can add a few drops of essential oils in a diffuser to get the advantage of therapeutic aromatherapy. There are different types of diffusers that you can choose from candle burners to lamp rings and water vapor diffusers. Heat may cause essential oils to degrade and evaporate quickly, and cold air diffusers should be preferred over heat diffusers. You can use different blends of diffusers together to create soothing effects and enjoy their health effects.

The essential oils work in a particular way because whenever you inhale an essential oil, the molecules of its odor may travel up to the nose allied to the nerves of the olfactory membranes in the nose. These molecules can excite the inside layer of nerve cells and enhance the electrical impulses to the olfactory bulb of your brain. This particular part of your brain transmits the impulses to the amygdala. The amygdala is the place where the memories are usually stored, and connected to the limbic system of the brain.

There is a direct connection between the limbic system and the other parts of your brain. These parts of your brain are responsible for controlling the heart rate, breathing, blood pressure, memory, stress level and hormones. The aroma of essential oils can excite the release of hormones and alter the behavior of your body and mind. The fragrance and unique molecular structure of the essential oils can stimulate the limbic lobe. You can inhale essential oils to reduce stress and emotional shock. You can trigger the production of thyroid hormones and other important hormones to improve your health and increase your life.

Emotional Brain Give Response to Smell Only

Amygdala is an important part of the brain that plays a significant role in treating emotional shocks. The scents of essential oils directly linked to the emotional states and behavior of a person. Smell is one of the five senses with a direct connection to the emotional control center. It can gradually overcome the fear, anger, anxiety, depression and all negative emotions.

You can learn about calming blends to promote your sleep, reduce stress and anxiety and enhance your mood. This book has lots of things for you to discover.

Chapter 1 – Amazing Essential Oil Diffusers for Sleep

There are lots of essential oils that can help you to relieve the symptoms of stress, anxiety and depression and enjoy a sound sleep. You can treat your anxiety with the use of some scented essential oils. A right scent will make you happy; therefore, you should select a scent carefully. Following are some essential oils that can help you to get rid of tension and depression:

- **Basil Essential Oil:** It can enhance your mood and work to remove emotions of anxiety, fatigue and depress.

- **Clary Safe Essential Oil:** It is an excellent essential oil to get rid of insomnia, tension, anxiety, and depression.

- **Frankincense:** If you are suffering from stress, anxiety, fear and tension, then you should use this essential oil to slow down these emotions.

- **Geranium Essential Oil:** It may reduce your stress and depression because it naturally works to enhance the spirit and release the negative emotions out.

- **Jasmine Essential Oil:** It is a relaxing and an antispasmodic essential oil with mood-lifting properties.

- **Lemon Essential Oil:** The refreshing scent of the lemon essential oil can enhance your mood. It enables you to fight with the stress, negative emotions, and depression.

- **Mandarin Essential Oil:** The antispasmodic properties help you to uplift the spirit.

- **Marjoram:** If you are feeling grief, fear, rejection, anxiety, and loneliness, then this is an excellent essential oil to enhance your mood.

- **Wild Orange:** It is good to increase your energy and enhance your mood. It is excellent to relieve the feelings of anger, irritation, and nervousness.

- **Palmarosa:** It is excellent for the treatment of nervous tension and anxiety.

- **Rose:** It can stimulate the sense of well-being by treating tension and nervousness.

- **Roman Chamomile:** It is ideal to relax your body and mind. It is an ultimate treatment for the depression and stress.

- **Sandalwood:** Its scent has magical properties to relieve tension and stress.

- **Ylang-Ylang:** The relaxing scent of ylang-ylang is equally good to energize both men and women. The scent of this essential oil can increase your confidence and treat depression, insomnia, and stress.

BLENDS
for sleep!

6 Drops RutaVaLa

4 Drops Lavender
4 Drops Peace & Calming

4 Drops Lavender
3 Drops Bergamot

4 Drops Frankincense
3 Drops Vetiver

2 Drops Lavender
2 Drops Cedarwood
2 Drops Peace & Calming

3 Drops Lavender
3 Drops Roman Chamomile
1 Drop Vetiver

2 Drops Lavender
2 Drops Vetiver
2 Drops Valerian
2 Drops Orange

4 Drops Lavender
1 Drop Bergamot
1 Drop Patchouli
1 Drop Ylang Ylang

Essential Oils for Loneliness

Isolation and loneliness are not good for anyone because it can harm you because during isolation, your mind filled with lots of negative thoughts and emotions. You prefer to live in isolation, but during the adverse times, it is important to take the help of your friends and love. The Ayurveda offers the best solution and it is meditation. You can talk to God during medication and offer a small prayer to comfort yourself. This will bring a great difference in your condition. There are some essential oils that will give you the energy to fight with the loneliness and support your mind.

Special Blend for Loneliness

If you are feeling lonely, then try this blend to get power for your mind and body:

- Rose oil

- Chamomile oil

- Frankincense oil

- Clary sages oil

- Bergamot oil

Take 1 to 2 drops of the oils and add into your bathtub to take a bath. You need to use a diffuser to reduce the intensity of the oils. You can use olive oil or almond oil as a carrier oil to defuse the blend. It will be good to apply this blend on your handkerchief and keep it with you to get energy and power to fight lonesomeness.

Note: The helichrysum and palo santo essential oils are also good to treat loneliness.

Chapter 2 – Get Rid of Stress and Anxiety with Essential Oil Diffusers

If you are dealing with anxious feelings, then it is important to use essential oils because these are better to use as compared to medicines. Following are some essential oils that you can use to treat your anxiety:

Balance Essential Oil

This essential oil is a blend of rosewood, blue tansy, spruce, and frankincense. It is an ideal essential oil to treat your anxiety. You can get a feeling of calmness with the use of this oil. It is a natural remedy used to calm down your nerves and promote the relaxation. The chamomile is used to soothe your nerves. The Frankincense can promote your relaxation and relieve the feelings of sorrow.

Lavender Essential Oil

If you are dealing with anxiousness, then you can try the lavender essential oil. Its scent is really calm and attractive, and you can use it in the water while taking a bath. You can also add it few drops in the deodorant to make it relaxing. There is a number of scientific proves that the lavender can reduce the anxiety and enhance the mood of patients.

Wild Orange Essential Oils

Wild orange essential oil is a great choice to reduce anxiety and boost your mood. It can increase your happiness and well-being. It is not good to eat any essential oil, but you can add a few drops of orange essential oils in your recipe to enhance citrus flavor.

Serenity Essential Oil

Serenity is a useful essential oil prepared to treat your anxiety. You can combine this essential oil with the lavender, sweet marjoram, ylang-ylang, sandalwood, and vanilla. These all oils have excellent properties, and you can enjoy a massage of these oils to promote sleep. The ylang-ylang is really beneficial for your central nervous system. The serenity can be applied topically or you may diffuse it in the air. You can apply it to the bottom of your feet before going to bed to enjoy a deep and relaxing sleep.

Bergamot Essential Oil

The bergamot is used to relieve the tension and stress, and it can also be used to improve the health of your skin. It features citrus scent and you can use it to enhance your mood. The bergamot can promote the relaxation by reducing the feelings of anxiousness. It is the best essential oil to apply to the skin or diffuse in the air to treating the tension and promote a good sleep. In order to enhance the benefits of essential oils, it will be good to use magnesium supplement to overcome your anxious feelings.

Grounding Blend

It is a useful blend of howood, spruce, frankincense and chamomile. If you are suffering from anxiety and tension, then this blend will really help you. It can promote the feelings of calmness and reduce your stress.

Application:

The grounding blend can be applied to your feet on a regular basis. You can also massage it over the back of your neck, heart and the wrists get better results.

Apply on the wrists and rub them together and inhale. You can mix this oil with a calming blend to increase its benefits.

Respiratory Blend

It is a versatile blend used for all respiratory issues. It is a combination of peppermint, lemon, ravensara lead, melaleuca and Cardamom seeds. It will help you to calm down your brain during anxiety.

Application:

Apply a few drops on your chest to relax your nerves and open your airways for relaxed breathing.

Frankincense

It is a king of essential oils that is why it is really valuable to slow down the fear, anxiety and tension. If you are suffering from stressful feelings, then it is an excellent choice for you. It can help you to combat the feelings of fear and anxiety.

Directions:

It is a great oil for regular use because it can promote your cellular balance. It can reduce feelings of anxiety, so use it in the diffuse state. You can inhale it, or massage your feet and back with a few drops of oil. Blend of lavender oil and wild orange can help you to get rid of anxiety.

Try a Joyful Blend

The smell of this oil will be great to treat the feelings of anxiety and tensions. It can treat anxiety and depression at the same time. The blend contains lavender, tangerine, elemi, lemon, Melissa, ylang-ylang, sandalwood, and osmanthus.

Directions:

You can apply it on your heart, bones, behind the ear, neck, forehead and wrists to reduce stress. Its regular application will help you to calm your mind and get rid of tensions.

Lemon Essential Oil

It is a versatile oil with lots of benefits because of its properties. The lemon oil is excellent to uplift your mood, revive your stressful feelings, and stimulate your feelings. The lemon enhances the sense of security and trust. It can help you to remove confusions and tensions. It can clear the obstacles and improve your feelings.

Directions:

You can use it on a regular basis in water. Just add 1 drop of essential oil in a glass of water and then use it for the whole day.

Calming Blend

If you want to promote relaxed feelings, then this blend is excellent for you. It can control your anger and promote good health with calmness. The blend contains sweet marjoram, lavender, ylang-ylang, roman chamomile, sandalwood, and vanilla bean.

Direction:

Use almost 5 drops of this blend in the hot water for relaxation. You can also apply it on the back of your neck and inhale it through a diffuser. Some drops should be applied to the bottoms of your feet before going to sleep. Awesome smell can leave excellent effects on your nerves.

Patchouli Essential Oil

It is a special oil to harmonize your mind and keep it stable without any tension. It can reduce the negative thoughts by relieving the depression and increase the joy in your life. You can recover from tension, stress and tiredness of mind.

Direction:

You can apply a diffused form of this oil to the base of your skull. Inhale the aroma of the oil to calm your fortitude and reduce disorganized thoughts.

Woody Diffuser for Calming Effects

Cypress oil: 2 drops

White first oil: 2 drops

Wintergreen oil: 2 drops

Spiced Chai

Cardamom oil: 3 drops

Cassia oil: 2 drops

Clove oil: 2 drops

Ginger oil: 1 drop

Enjoy Autumn Smell

Wild orange oil: 3 drops

Cinnamon bark oil: 2 drops

Clove oil: 1 drop

Calming Effects

Frankincense oil: 3 drops

White fir oil: 2 drops

Cedarwood oil: 1 drop

Boost Immunity

Rosemary oil: 1 drop

Clove oil: 1 drop

Cinnamon bark oil: 1 drop

Eucalyptus oil: 1 drop

Wild orange oil: 1 drop

Stress Buster Blend

Frankincense oil: 2 drops

Bergamot oil: 2 drops

Enhance Sleep

Lavender oil: 2 drops

Chamomile oil: 2 drops

Vetiver essential oil: 2 drops

Chapter 3 – Essential Oil Diffusers to Enhance Happiness

Everyone has its own reasons to become happy, but if you want to increase your joy, then you should use some essential oils. These oils can help you to enhance the joy in your life. There are lots of uses of these essential oils, such as you can increase your joy and happiness of your party by diffusing few oils. You can also memorize the days of winter holidays by using Cinnamon, Ginger, and a little Orange essential oil. Put a few drops of these oils in the evaporator to increase the happiness. The blend of various oils will be a unique way to enhance your mood. Some blends of essential oils help women to stabilize their hormones. The blend will only help women without affecting the hormonal balance of another person in the house. Following are some essential oils that will help you to increase your happiness.

Bergamot Essential Oil

The fresh, citrus oil and refreshing scent of the essential oils can uplift your mood. The aroma of this oil will help you to feel bright, happy and energized. It is excellent for your healthy skin and improve good health. It is useful for its antiseptic properties, particularly for the skin that is prone to acne. It is useful for eczema and other conditions that can increase stress.

Geranium Essential Oil

This is an excellent essential oil to harmonize, comfort, calm and balance your mood. It can uplift your mood and strengthen your mind to get rid of tensions and anxiety. It is a wonderful oil for skin care and treat menopause condition as well. The oil is equally good to use for a healthy and excellent skin. If you have dry and oily skin, you can use it because of its antiseptic and anti-inflammatory properties. It can heal the reasons of tension and uplift your mood.

Enhance Happiness

Wild orange: 2 drops

Wintergreen oil: 2 drops

Boost Your Mood

Wild orange oil: 2 drops

Frankincense oil: 2 drops

Cinnamon oil: 2 drops

Chillout Essential Oil

Vetiver essential oil: 2 drops

Cedarwood essential oil: 2 drops

Happy Diffuser Oil

Wild orange: 2 drops

White fir: 2 drops

Wintergreen: 1 drop

Chapter 4 – Essential Oil Diffusers to Manage Anger

There are lots of essential oils that can help you to relax. The strong aroma of these oils will relax your nerves and help you to control negative emotions. Following are some essential oils that are really beneficial for your health:

Peace and Calming Blend

You can prepare a blend of orange, tangerine, ylang-ylang, blue tansy and patchouli because this blend is excellent to manage your anger. It can promote the feelings of peace and reduce your stress level.

Directions:

If you want to treat your anger, then you should consider this blend because the massage of this oil will help you to manage anger. Use it in a diffused state and promote peace and calmness. Add a drop of oil in your bath water, or you can use it as a perfume as well.

Ylang Ylang

It is an excellent essential oil used in a diffused form to treat anger. The properties of this special essential oil will help you to reduce anxiety, blood pressure, frustration and much more.

Directions:

If you want to take the benefits of this essential oil, then apply it on your feet in a diffused form. You can also rub it on your spin on your lower back to get rid of anger.

Roman Chamomile Essential Oil

If an angry outburst is an important part of your conversation, then you should try this essential oil. This oil has magical properties to treat allergy, cleanse your blood, calm your sorrow and grieves.

Directions:

You can apply this essential oil on your throat in a diffused form. It will help you to stabilize your anger and bring your emotions to a balance.

Lavender Essential Oil

The lavender is famous for its soothing and calming properties because after its application, you can feel relaxed. It can treat allergies, digestion problems; reduce nausea and many other problems. Its regular massage will promote your good health and enhance your mood.

Directions:

The lavender can be inhaled from the bottle, or you can rub the back of your neck after taking this oil on your hands. It will help you to reduce stress and tension. The oil has excellent properties to diffuse your anger.

Geranium Essential Oil

This is an excellent essential oil, and you should include it in your daily routine. The essential oil is excellent to make your skin beautiful and support your circulatory and nervous system. It is excellent to invigorate your body tissues.

Directions:

You can use this oil to promote brain health, and it is quite easy to use because it is good to inhale it directly. Few drops of diffused geranium essential oil can be rubbed on your neck to get rid of anger.

Sandalwood Essential Oil

The sandalwood essential oil can treat your emotional issues, relieve stress and unwind the tensions. Aloes are its other name, and you can rub your backbone, wrist, and neck with the help of diffused sandalwood essential oil. This oil is really good for your skin. After its frequent use, you can be able to get rid of all tensions and anger emotions.

Blue Tansy Essential Oil

It has slightly sweet aroma and used to manage anger. If you are suffering from anger and other negative emotions, then use this essential oil because it has lots of benefits. The famous species of tansy plants are Moroccan and Chamomile.

Directions:

- Take a few drops of diffused essential oil, and apply it on your feet. It can calm your mind and alleviate the negative emotions.

- You can also add a few drops in your bath to promote the feelings of relaxation.

Soothing Blends:

Following are some blends that will help you to promote the feelings of relaxation and enhance your mood:

Blend 01:

- 1 drop Rose

- 3 drops Orange

- 1 drop Vetiver

Mix all these essential oils and pour it in the water before taking a bath. It will help you to reduce anger.

Blend 02:

- 3 drops Bergamot

- 1 drop Ylang Ylang

- 1 drop Jasmine

Add this blend to your bath water and take a bath with it to gradually reduce your anger.

Blend 03:

- 1 drop Roman Chamomile

- 2 drops Bergamot

- 2 Drops Orange Essential Oil

Take a relaxing bath after adding this blend in a bucket of water, and get the benefits of this bath.

Blend 04:

- 3 drops of Orange Essential Oil

- 2 drops of Patchouli Oil

This will be the relaxing blend for to manage your anger. Include it in a bucket of water to take a bath or add it in a diffuser to keep it in your room

Tips to Diffuse Your Blend

You can increase the amount of blend by adding your oil in a dark colored bottle made of glass and then roll the bottle between your hands. You can add a diffuser like olive oil to diffuse the blend and use this blend in your bath water.

Carrier Oils

The carrier oils are often used as a diffuser to diffuse the intensity of carrier oils. You can mix these oils with essential oils to take aromatherapy. Following are some famous and frequently used carrier oils:

- Sweet almond oil

- Olive oil

- Sunflower oil

In short, the seed, vegetable, and nut oils can be used to dilute the concentrated essential oils.

Rose Essential Oils

The rose essential oils are famous for its properties because it can be used as an antidepressant, antiseptic, antispasmodic, hepatic, uterine, stomachic, etc. The rose essential oil works well to alleviate stress, mental tension, depression, nervous ailments and various other problems. If you want to get rid of anger and mental stress, then use rose essential oil to manage this situation.

Palo Santo Essential Oil

The palo santo essential oil is used to manage anger because its scent can keep your mind free from worries and tensions. Its anti-inflammatory properties can help you to avoid cancer as well. The regular use of this oil will help you to manage anger and stress.

Diffuser

- 5 drops Cedarwood Atlas

- 4 drops Palo Santo

- 1 drop Patchouli

- 5 drops of Bergamot

Bug Repellent Diffuser of Essential Oil

Lemongrass oil: 1 drop

Thyme oil: 1 drop

Eucalyptus oil: 1 drop

Basil oil: 1 drop

Chapter 5 – Increase Your Confidence with Essential Oil Diffusers

There are lots of essential oils that are used during performing religious traditions. The exotic fragrance and purities of the essential oil can improve your mood. There are a number of essential oils that can be used to increase self-confidence.

Cypress Essential Oil

The cypress essential oil is famous for its properties because it can help you to treat lots of problems. It can help you to extricate stuck emotions. If you are feeling any tension and want to ignore everything, then push things aside and shove negative emotions. The negative emotions make it really hard to feel relaxed and the cypress can help you to bring an accurate balance to your mind and spirit. You can get rid of fear and treat your negative emotions with the help of cypress essential oil.

Directions:

You can use it in diluted form and then massage several locations of your body. You should consider the vita flex points to get optimum benefits.

Peppermint Essential Oils

If you want to enhance your energy and confidence, then the peppermint essential oil will be an excellent drug for you. There is no need to drink caffeine because the essential oil can increase your energy levels. The peppermint oil trickles the freshness and improves your mental health. It can keep you alert and enables you to tackle each task in a better way.

Directions:

Peppermint essential oil can uplift your mood and confidence. You can include a few drops of peppermint oil in your bath water to keep your mind fresh. It will reduce tension, anxiety and enhance the feelings of calmness. In the absence of tension and anxiety, you can perform in a better way.

Sandalwood Essential Oil

If you have dry or irritated skin, then you may feel low in the public places because a smooth and beautiful skin can boost your confidence. With dull and dry skin, you will only think about the negative views of people about you. If you want a glowing and healthy skin, then you should add a few drops of sandalwood essential oil in your body lotion. It will make your skin healthy and increase its glow. When you feel good in your own skin, your self-confidence will be at a higher level.

Bergamot Essential Oil

The bergamot essential oil is an excellent addition to your daily routine because it can improve the health of your skin. It is often used in the production of perfumes and has amazing healing powers. This oil is equally good for your brain because it can cure your stress, tension, and anger in a better way. If you want to increase your self-confidence, you should reduce your stress, anxiety, and tension. The Bergamot essential oil will play an important role in this.

Rosemary Essential Oil

If you want to boost your confidence, then you should focus on your personal improvement. The rosemary essential oil will increase the shine and smooth texture of your hair. Just add five drops of rosemary oil in the bottle of shampoo. It will make your hair silky and keep your scalp free from dandruff. If you are suffering from migraines, then instead of using tablets, try this oil. Use a drop of this oil and massage on your wrists. Take q few deep breaths and feel the calm sensation.

Tea Tree Essential Oil

If you are feeling any problem just because of virus and bacteria around you, then you should use tea tree oil. The oil will serve as a body bouncer and improve the immune system of your body in a natural way. It will save your money because after using this, there is no need to use expensive treatments. You can pamper your skin with the help of this oil because it may reduce the acne from your skin. Tea tree oil will be an ultimate solution of your all problems. Take a bath by adding a few drops of tea tree essential oils in water.

Chamomile Essential Oil

It is quite surprising to know that the chamomile is an excellent mood booster. If you are feeling burdened and want to get rid of these feelings, then use this oil. Just add a few drops of chamomile oil in the boiling water, and take a bath to see its magic.

Ylang-Ylang Essential Oil

If you have ylang-ylang essential oil, then you can turn your own bathroom into a spa by adding a few drops of this oil in water. This will help you to control your emotions, and you may feel relaxed. This essential oil is available in a small bottle, and you can use it in different ways. If you don't want to take a bath, then you can add a few drops in a very small bottle and spray this water on your face. It will enhance the feelings of calmness and relaxation. This is an excellent mood booster and increases your self-confidence as well.

There are lots of powerful essential oils that can increase your self-confidence and enhance your mood. You can inhale these oils or take a bath by adding a few drops. If you want to enjoy enough benefits of essential oils, then find the right oil for you to restore your energy. It will increase your self-confidence by boosting your mood.

Diffuser to Increase Your Alertness

Wild orange oil: 2 drops

Peppermint oil: 2 drops

Fresh Diffuser of Essential Oil

Lavender oil: 2 drops

Lemon oil: 2 drops

Rosemary oil: 2 drops

Odor Eliminator

Lemon oil: 2 drops

Melaleuca oil: 1 drop

Cilantro oil: 1 drop

Lime oil: 1 drop

Seasonal Diffuser

Lavender oil: 2 drops

Lemon oil: 2 drops

Peppermint oil: 2 drops

Citrus Explosion Oil

Lemon oil: 1 drop

Wild orange oil: 2 drops

Lime oil: 1 drop

Grapefruit oil: 1 drop

Deep Breath Essential Oil Diffusers

Bergamot oil: 1 drop

Patchouli oil: 1 drop

Ylang ylang oil: 1 drop

Respiratory Blend

Lemon oil: 1 drop

Eucalyptus oil: 1 drop

Peppermint oil: 2 drops

Rosemary oil: 1 drop

Flower Garden Diffuser

Lavender oil: 2 drops

Geranium oil: 1 drop

Roman Chamomile oil: 2 drops

Precautionary Tips for Essential Oil

It is really good to use essential oils, but you have to consider safety and effectiveness. Following are some general guideline and precautions that will help you:

- You need to keep essential oils away from the reach of children and pets.

- The essential oils with high menthol like peppermint should not be used on the throat and neck of the children under 30 months.

- The essential oils can't dilute in the water; therefore, you can mix them in the vegetable oil to dissolve in water.

- The oils are available in the concentrated state; therefore, you should use them in diluted form. The concentrated oil should not come in contact with the sensitive skin areas.

- Undiluted oils should not be directly poured into the bath water.

- If you have sensitive skin, then the oil should not be applied directly on the skin. Dilute it with a carrier oil and then apply to the neat and clean soles of the feet.

- If you have allergies, then you should be careful while using essential oils. The sole of your feet is the least sensitive area, and you can apply oil on the sole.

- Some essential oils have strong caustic properties; dilute these essential oils before using them.

- Some citrus essential like orange, lemon and bergamot and petitgrain should not be applied directly on the skin if you have to go out. These oils are phototoxic and you need to avoid direct sunlight for almost 48hours.

- Before trying any kind of essential oil, you need to do a patch test of the diluted oil to know if it is irritating you.

- A number of essential oils are not good to ingest; therefore, you have to be careful. Properly know the properties of the essential oils before ingesting them. It is good to take the advice of your health care advisor before consuming any oil.

- If you have sensitive skin, heart and kidney problems, asthma, and other serious medical conditions, then you should consult your doctor for the safety of any essential oil for you.

- The properties of essential oil can't be judged on the basis of the properties of its plants.

- Keep the essential oils away from heat, flame, and all ignition sources.

- You need to be careful while applying essential oils on the skin because some personal care products may contain synthetic and petrochemicals. These can penetrate and remain in the skin and fatty tissues for various days. The essential oils can react with these chemicals to cause irritation, nausea, and other displeasures.

- There can be a strong reaction of essential oils on the body because of the chemicals in food, water, and the environment. If your skin gets any reaction, then stop the use of essential oil and start internal cleansing before resuming to the regular routine. You can increase the water intake to reduce any adverse reaction.

Precautions for An Accident with Essential Oils

If an essential oil falls into your eyes accidentally, the immediately flush it with cold milk or vegetable oil to dilute the oil. If you still feel any stinging, you can consult a doctor immediately.

You can use cream or vegetable oil to remove the additional essential oils from your skin. Use soap and warm water to remove additional oil from the skin.

If you ingest any essential oil accidently, then you can call national poison control center for assistance.

Conclusion

Essential oils can affect your mind and emotions in a better way because of their strong scent. The aromas of essential oils can have a good impact on your emotions, and can reach deep into the psyche. It can keep your mind relaxed and uplift your spirit. You will be amazed to know that the smelling sense of human beings is 10,000 times more sensitive than other senses.

The scents can travel at a faster rate to the brain and improve your sound and sight at the same time. It is better to use essential oils for your emotions as compared to medicines. There are lots of side effects directly linked to the medications, but the essential oils have no side-effects.

The essential oils work in a particular way because whenever you inhale an essential oil, the molecules of its odor may travel up to the nose allied to the nerves of the olfactory membranes in the nose. These molecules can excite the inside layer of nerve cells and enhance the electrical impulses to the olfactory bulb of your brain. This particular part of your brain transmits the impulses to the amygdala. The amygdala is the place where the memories are usually stored, and connected to the limbic system of the brain.

30 Summer & Spring Essential Oil Diffuser Recipes

Introduction

Essential oils play a significant role in carrying out our routine activities without any hurdle and without facing any kind of ambiguity. As you know that these oils are just the extracts of different kinds of herbs and are used for fulfilling many kinds of purposes.

The essence of these herbs and plants is very useful in a way that in case you opt for dried herbs for any purpose, a huge quantity of them is required in comparison to few drops of essential oils. These oils are naturally present in the herbs and plants and not only is their individual effect of worth consideration.

Just like all other essential oils, frankincense oil has also got the ability of providing you with ultimate health benefits and it is also used widely as diffusers. This book is all about the best uses of frankincense essential oil diffusers and the ways by which you can use them during summers and winters.

Importance of essential oils as diffusers cannot be denied. So, you can use them without any difficulty and without any fear of side effects. In this book, I am going to tell you the importance of the natural essential oil diffusers along with some of the diffuser recipes which you should try in order to get your work done. If you are thinking that you may get any sort of side effects by using these oils then I must say, do not worry about the side effects at all.

Chapter 1 – An introduction to essential oil diffusers

Essential oils are very much beneficial for you if you use them for useful purposes. In the modern era when people prefer to use latest medicines and technology based treatments for getting better health, there are also present many herbal treatments as well which will help you out in getting rid of any problem you have. There are certain natural essential oils as well which can be matter if you are having any sort of skin problem or your hair are suffering from dryness, essential oils of every kind are avail which will assist you in getting flawless beauty and beautiful hair.

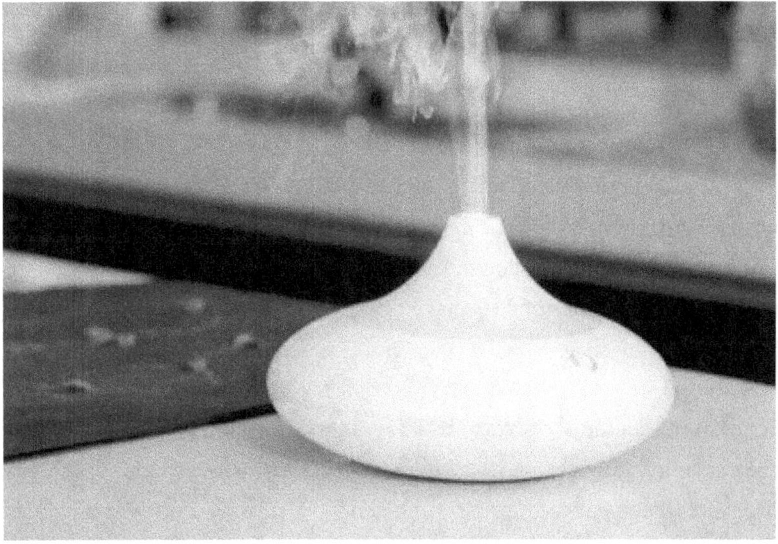

Just a little drop of natural oil at a time can bring calmness, can help us to focus on various things which are required, can help in reducing the tensions which we face. It can help in calming down our muscles, in making our digestion better and to make use physically and mentally strong to face the day to day challenges which come to our way.

Various combinations of essential oils in different kinds of recipes are also very much beneficial for the users. Just like all other essential oils, natural essential oil also helps you a lot in gaining extravagant benefits. There are so many uses of this essential oil and following are the main reasons why the natural oil is used in a variety of ways.

We are living a life where we are completely surrounded by numerous kinds of chemicals which are definitely not healthy for us and they are eventually making us sick. Like the detergents, soaps, air fresheners and numerous other things are there which are a part of our everyday life and are just adding negative impacts on our wellbeing.

While we are surrounded by so many unnatural harmful products, we are in need of using something which should grant us with unmatchable health benefits in a natural way. The essential oils prove to be so much beneficial in this regard. Without any doubt, essential oils are having ideal solutions in a natural way for the harmful effects.

It has been thousands of years for the essential oils are in use of humans and are providing ultimate and matchless benefits in many aspects. These oils have got therapeutic properties and are greatly used in the practice of aromatherapy as these oils are having some healing properties as well. The main source of essential oils is stems, leaves and roots of plants from where they are extracted.

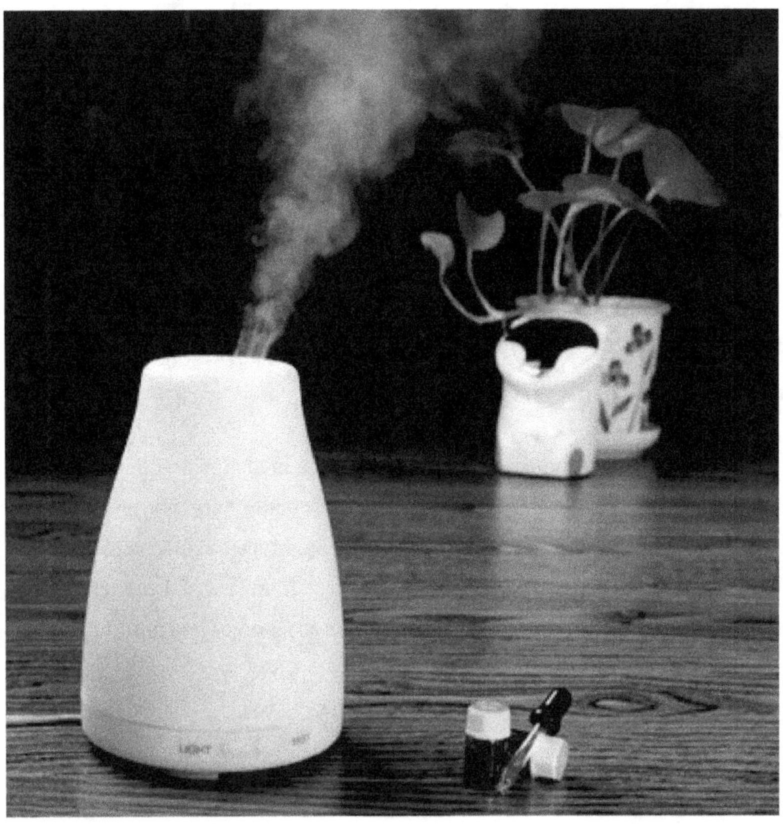

In the modern era, the lifestyle of people has seen a dramatic change. It can proved to be full of stress at many times but this stress can be taken away by one way or the other. In modern times, people are addicted to technology and the recent milestones which have been achieved by the scientists, but we cannot neglect this fact that the herbal and natural remedies which have been used by our ancestors cannot be overlooked at any cost.

These natural remedies from natural extracts have got so much power that they can make us feel better by one way or the other. It has been in practice since very long ago when generations after generations, people used to have the natural ingredients to make their life better. Despite of having so much latest medicines and technology in the modern era, the importance of those herbal extracts and their use in making the life better cannot be denied.

Today just like other things, the use of essential oils is also having so much significance and demand that no one can deny. In fact, these essential oils can be used not only for curing many kinds problems related to health but also helps in getting out of that problem without any side effects.

Since very long ago, the use of essential oils as a medicine and in many other aspects have been continued and they are actually very powerful natural agents which are being used for curing various types of problems and till present day the importance of these chemical free essential oils cannot be denied in any case. You can also use these oils as summer and spring diffusers with much ease.

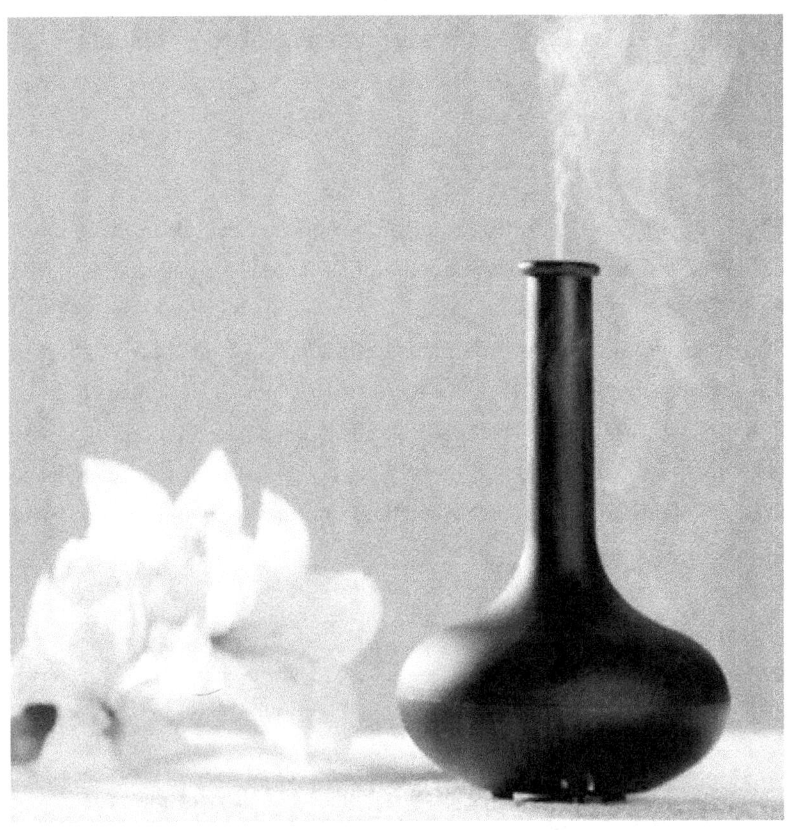

All of these essential oils are free of any chemicals which can proved to be harmful for your health. So, you can have use of all of these natural essential oil diffusers while keeping your eye even closed. In presence of so many modern techniques, essential oil's use cannot be deigned and if you want to get immense benefits out of it, you must use them as per the instructions as I am going to tell you. The main benefit of using these essential oils diffusers is that they can be used without any risk of getting any harm because they are free of any chemicals and harmful ingredients.

Chapter 2 – Why to opt for natural essential oil diffusers?

The herbs which are used for the extraction of essential oils are very much beneficial and are being in use for centuries. The oils are mostly extracted from the herbs and plants and are used for multiple purposes. The essential oils are extracted from various origins like orange peel, lemon peel, almond, lavender, eucalyptus etc. There is a much wider exposure of humans to these essential oils which are chemical free. The main benefit of using these essential oils for the treatment of anything is that these oils are completely deprived of any harmful or side effect thus you can use them in any way and for getting anything cured.

Exceptional properties

Not only this, but many of the essential oils have also got the property of having extra ordinary fragrance, so these oils can also be used as a fragrance and a very good example of such a fragrance is the rose essential oil, which is not only used for the tremens of various skin problems but also used as a fragrance and as an essential part of many concentrated perfumes.

Thus we can say that the essential oils have got immense importance which cannot be denied in any case and if you want to get all the bandits out of these oils you must follow all the steps and techniques of using the essential oils for treatment of any problem.

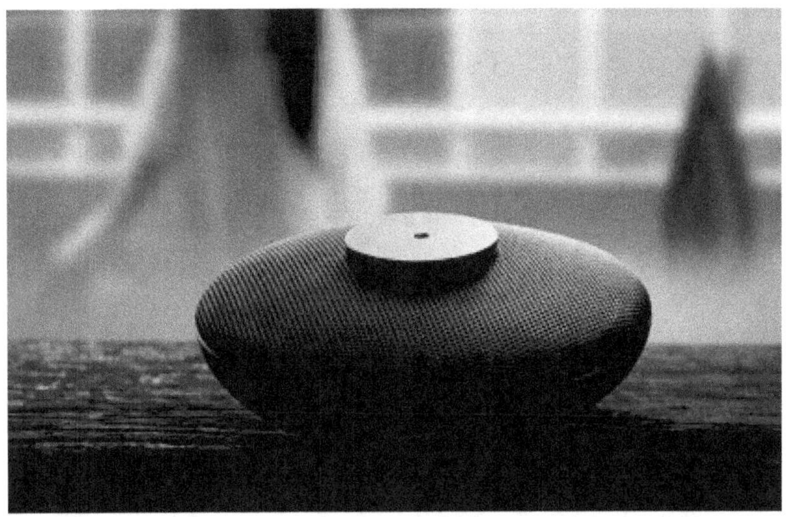

As far as the extent of choosing the right oils are concerned for making right fragrance, it is basically up to you that what kind of fragrance do you like and what are those ingredients which you want to be added as an essential component of deodorant you are making. Sometimes, you cannot become able to decide what to do with the ingredients you have. But do not worry at all as I have given the exact and perfect combination of different oils so that different types of fragrances can be made out of them.

The idea behind choosing the diffusers which I will be giving you in the coming chapters lies in the fact that I was thinking about different occasions where some kind of festivity or joy will be or different types of mood which I may have depending upon the environment in which I am present. So, you must be having the same thinking for sure as for different occasions you will be having different moods as well.

The diffusers which are manufactured synthetically can be composed of some harmful chemicals which can harm your skin and which should not be taken in to your consideration when you are looking for some diffuser in any local store near you. So, you are just in a need of having some organic essential oils so that you can use them without facing any problem.

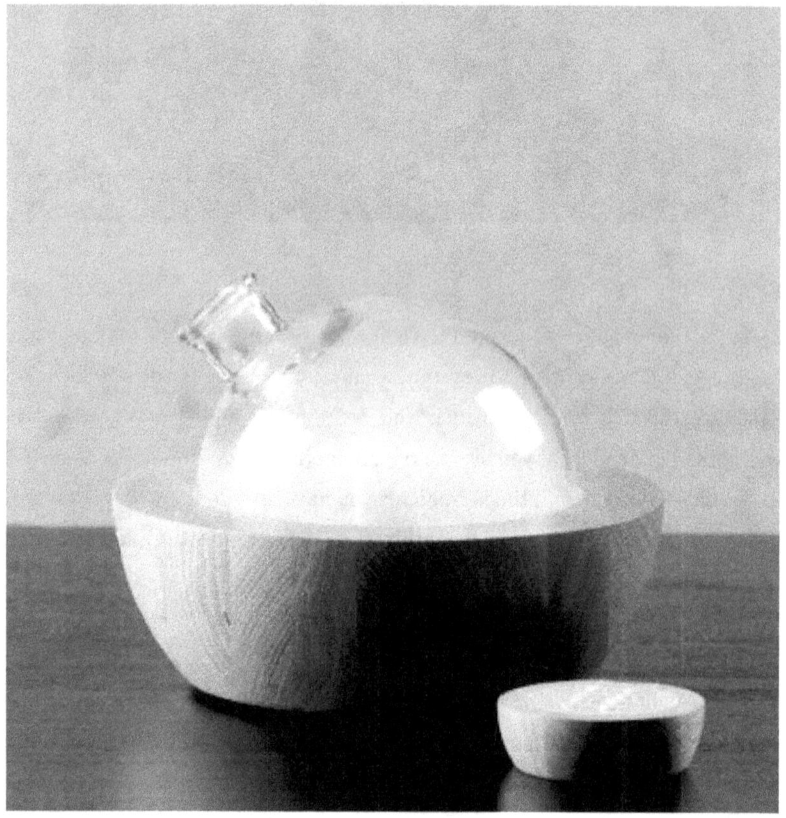

One important aspect of homemade diffuser is that, you can have their fragrance with you for quite a longer period of time, sometimes for all day, unlike that of synthetic diffusers who may disappear just after some time.

It is true that all of us having a desire of smelling something good which is good in fragrance and which is liked by everyone. If you get to have your own diffuser of your own then it will really be that thing full of fun for you when you will use it in routine at so many occasions and for so many reasons. This signature secret will make you able to have some unique value of yours as compared to the people who are around you as it is that smell that is exclusively being used by you and not by anyone else.

At this stage, you should not forget this in any case that when you are going to make your own diffuser with the help of organic ingredients, you should be patient enough to look for the right things to do. Do not do anything which can take you towards hurry and be there to exhibit patience as some diffuser require some days to get in to that consistency which you are desiring to have with you.

Chapter 3 – 20 essential oil diffuser recipes

Recipe no. 1

Ingredients:

- Jojoba oil three drops

- Almond oil four drops

- Jasmine essential oil four drops

Method:

- Take all the oils that have been mentioned in the detailed list of ingredients and their quantity above.

- Beware that you are taking the right quantity just according to what have been mentioned in the ingredients above.

- Leave the bottle for about four days in a dry place or you can also place it in the sun for four to four hours daily so that all the oils get mixed with each other with a high level of consistency.

- Then keep the bottle at a place with the lowest level of humidity.

Recipe no. 2

Ingredients:

- Honey three drops

- Jojoba oil three drops

- Carrot oil four drops

- Jasmine essential oil four drops

- Lemon oil three drops

Method:

- Take all the oils that have been mentioned in the detailed list of ingredients and their quantity above.

- Take a small bottle or container and add all the above-mentioned ingredients.

- Close the lid of the bottle and mix the oils very well.

- Leave the bottle for about four to three days so that all the oils get mixed with each other with a high level of consistency.

- Then keep the bottle in cool and dry place.

- Place the diffuser cap at the top of the bottle.

- Press the button to have its fumes out whenever you need.

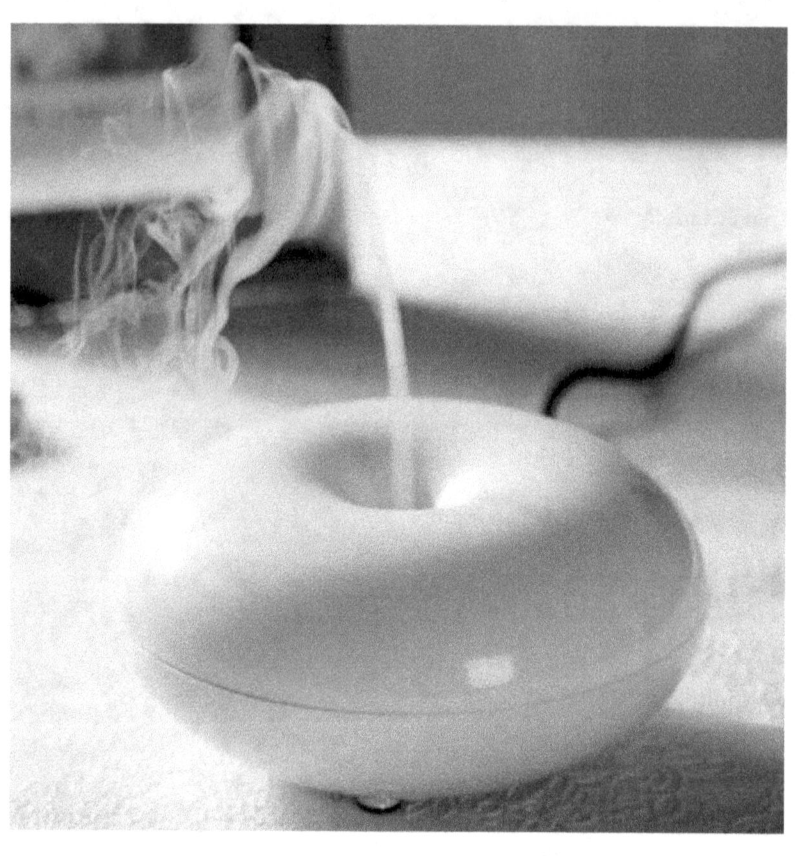

Recipe no. 3

Ingredients:

- Jojoba oil three drops

- Almond oil four drops

- Rose essential oil four drops

- Lemon oil four drops

Method:

- Take all the oils that have been mentioned in the detailed list of ingredients and their quantity above.

- Make the lid of the bottle closed and mix the oils well so that they can become smooth in consistency.

- Leave the bottle for about one day or 24 hours in a dry place or you can also place it in the sun for four to four hours daily so that all the oils get mixed with each other with a high level of consistency.

- Then keep the bottle at a place with the lowest level of humidity.

- Place the diffuser cap at the top of the bottle.

- Press the button to have its fumes out whenever you need.

Recipe no. 4

Ingredients:

- Lemon oil three drops

- Almond oil three drops

- Jojoba oil five drops

- Jasmine essential oil four drops

Method:

- Take all the oils that have been mentioned in the detailed list of ingredients and their quantity above.

- Take a small bottle or container and add all the ingredients that have been mentioned in the above-mentioned list for your convenience.

- Close the bottle's lid tightly so that no air can enter inside and mix all the mixtures well so that you can get the desired consistency out of it without any ambiguity on your way.

- Leave the bottle for about three to five days so that all the oils get mixed with each other with a high level of consistency.

- Place the diffuser cap at the top of the bottle.

- Press the button to have its fumes out whenever you need.

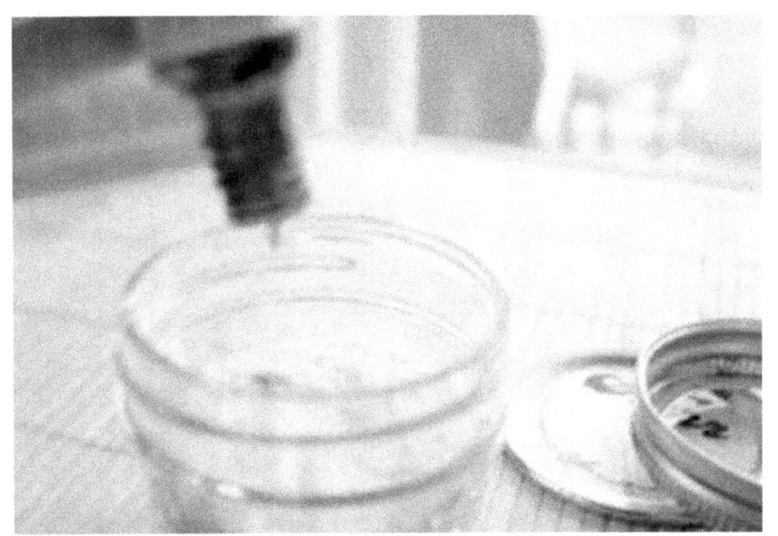

Recipe no. 5

Ingredients:

- Jojoba oil three drops

- Jasmine essential oil three drops

- Lemon oil four drops

- Almond oil four drops

Method:

- Take all the oils that have been mentioned in the detailed list of ingredients and their quantity above.

- Take a small bottle or container and add all the ingredients that have been mentioned in the above-mentioned list for your convenience.

- Make the lid of the bottle closed and mix the oils well so that they can become smooth in consistency.

- Now you should keep the bottle in dry place for about two to three days, so that all the ingredients get consistent.

- Place the diffuser cap at the top of the bottle.

- Press the button to have its fumes out whenever you need.

Recipe no. 6

Ingredients:

- Grapefruit oil three drops

- Jasmine essential oil four drops

- Sweet almond oil three drops

- Rose essential oil four drops

Method:

- Take all the oils that have been mentioned in the detailed list of ingredients and their quantity above.

- Beware that you are taking the right quantity just according to what have been mentioned in the ingredients above.

- Take a small bottle or container and add all the ingredients that have been mentioned in the above-mentioned list for your convenience.

- Leave the bottle for about four days in a dry place or you can also place it in the sun for four to four hours daily so that all the oils get mixed with each other with a high level of consistency.

- Place the diffuser cap at the top of the bottle.

- Press the button to have its fumes out whenever you need.

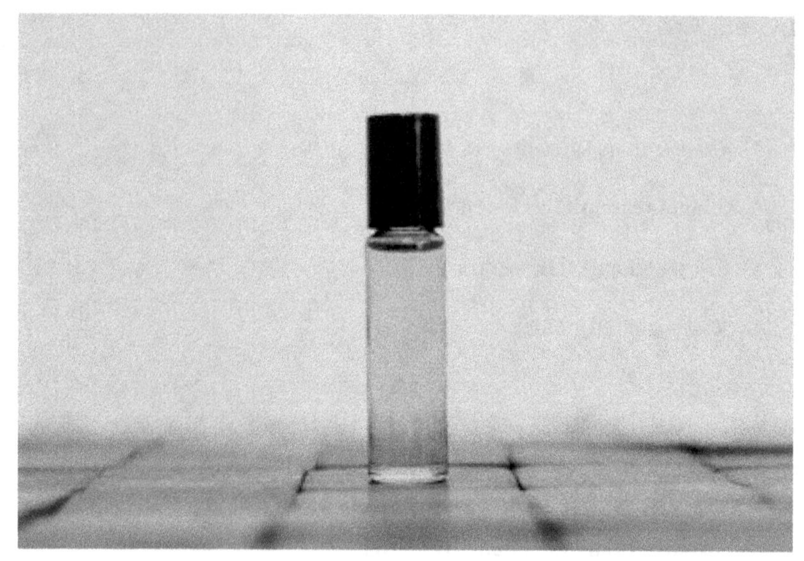

Recipe no. 7

Ingredients:

- Almond oil three drops

- Almond oil three drops

- Jasmine oil four drops

- Jasmine essential oil four drops

Method:

- Take all the oils that have been mentioned in the detailed list of ingredients.

- Beware that you are taking the right quantity as it is mentioned above.

- Take a small bottle or container and add all the ingredients that have been mentioned in the above-mentioned list for your convenience.

- Place the diffuser cap at the top of the bottle.

- Press the button to have its fumes out, whenever you need.

Recipe no. 8

Ingredients:

- Nutmeg oil three drops

- Rosemary oil four drops

- Jasmine essential oil four drops

- Almond oil four drops

- Black cumin oil four drops

Method:

- Take all the oils that have been above.

- Close the bottle's lid tightly so that no air can enter inside and mix all the mixtures well so that you can get the desired consistency out of it without any ambiguity on your way.

- Now you should keep the bottle in dry place for about two to three days, so that all the ingredients get consistent.

- Then keep the bottle in cool place.

- Place the diffuser cap at the top of the bottle.

- Press the button to have its fumes out whenever you need.

- Apply it to neck, back of year and wrist to get elegant fragrance.

Recipe no. 9

Ingredients:

- Lavender oil four drops

- Almond oil three drops

- Jojoba oil four drops

- Lemon oil three drops

Method:

- Take all the ingredients mentioned above in a small bottle with a cap.

- Beware that you are taking the right quantity just according to what have been mentioned in the ingredients above.

- Take a small bottle or container and add all the ingredients that have been mentioned in the above-mentioned list for your convenience.

- Now you should keep the bottle in dry place for about two to three days, so that all the ingredients get consistent.

- Place the diffuser cap at the top of the bottle.

- Press the button to have its fumes out whenever you need.

- Apply it to neck, back of year and wrist to get elegant fragrance.

Recipe no. 10

Ingredients:

- Almond oil three drops

- Cilantro oil four drops

- Jasmine essential oil 2 drops

Method:

- Take all the ingredients mentioned above in a small bottle with a cap.

- Beware that you are taking the right quantity as it is mentioned above.

- Close the bottle's lid tightly so that no air can enter inside and mix all the mixtures well.

- Place the diffuser cap at the top of the bottle.

- Press the button to have its fumes out whenever you need.

- Apply the body spray at the back of the ear, in front of neck, on the chest or at any place of your body where you are having the desire to apply it.

Recipe no. 11

Ingredients:

- Almond oil 3 teaspoon

- Lemon juice 3 drops

- Jasmine essential oil 3 drops

- Lemon oil 3 drops

Method:

- Take a small container and add all the ingredients that have been mentioned above.

- Close the cap of the container and mix the oils well.

- Leave the container for about 3 days so that the body spray can be enriched.

- Place the diffuser cap at the top of the bottle.

- Press the button to have its fumes out whenever you need.

- Apply the body spray at the back of the ear, in front of neck, or at any place of your body where you want.

Recipe no. 12

Ingredients:

- Rosemary oil 3 drops

- Almond oil 3 drops

- Raspberry essential oil 3 drops

- Jasmine essential oil 9 drops

Method:

- Take a small container and add all the ingredients that have been mentioned above.

- Make the cap of the bottle closed and mix the oils well so that they can become smooth in consistency.

- Leave the bottle for about 5 days in a dry place or you can also place it in the sun for 3 to 3 hours daily so that the body spray can be enriched.

- Then keep the bottle at a place with the lowest level of humidity.

- Place the diffuser cap at the top of the bottle.

- Press the button to have its fumes out whenever you need.

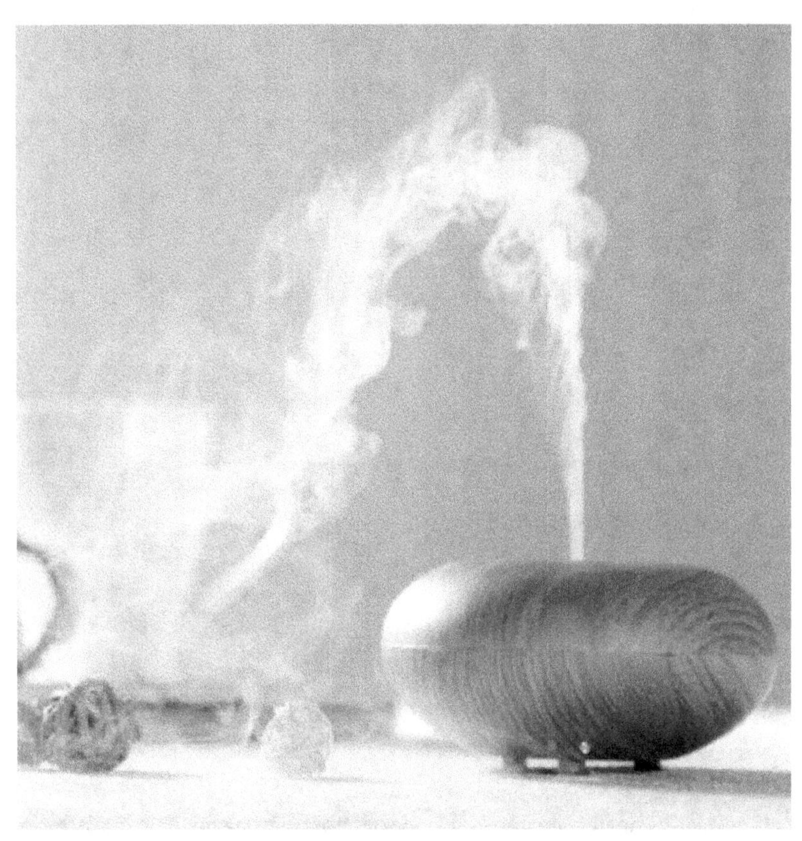

Recipe no. 13

Ingredients:

- Cumin oil 3 drops

- Ginger oil 3 drops

- Grapefruit oil 3 drops

- Jasmine essential oil 3 drops

- Raspberry essential oil 3 drops

Method:

- Take a small container and add all the ingredients that have been mentioned above.

- Close the bottle's cap tightly so that no air can enter inside and mix all the mixtures well so that you can get the desired consistency out of it without any ambiguity on your way.

- Leave the bottle for about 3 days so that the body spray can be enriched.

- Then keep the bottle in cool and dry place.

- Place the diffuser cap at the top of the bottle.

- Press the button to have its fumes out whenever you need.

Recipe no. 14

Ingredients:

* Rosemary oil 3 drops

* Almond oil 3 drops

* Raspberry essential oil 3 drops

* Jasmine essential oil 3 drops

Method:

* Take all the oils that have been mentioned in the detailed list of ingredients and their quantity above.

* Beware that you are taking the right quantity as it is mentioned above.

* Close the bottle's cap tightly so that no air can enter inside.

* Mix all the mixtures well so that you can get the desired consistency out of it.

* Then keep the bottle in cool and dry place.

* Place the diffuser cap at the top of the bottle.

* Press the button to have its fumes out whenever you need.

Recipe no. 15

Ingredients:

- Almond oil 3 drops

- Cilantro oil 3 drops

- Jasmine essential oil 3 drops

- Raspberry essential oil 3 drops

- Cumin oil 3 drops

Method:

- Take a small bottle or container and add all the ingredients that have been mentioned in the above-mentioned list for your convenience.

- Make the cap of the bottle closed and mix the oils well so that they can become smooth in consistency.

- Leave the bottle for about 3 days in a dry place or you can also place it in the sun for 3 to 3 hours daily so that the body spray can be enriched.

- Then keep the bottle at a place with the lowest level of humidity. Place the diffuser cap at the top of the bottle.

- Press the button to have its fumes out whenever you need.

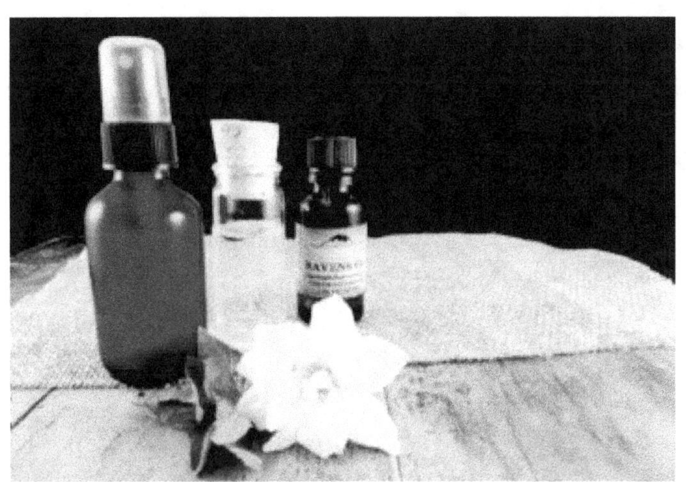

Recipe no. 16

Ingredients:

- Rose essential oil 3 drops

- Jasmine essential oil 3 drops

- Cumin oil 3 drops

- Lemon oil 3 drops

- Savory oil 3 drops

Method:

- Take a small bottle or container and add all the ingredients that have been mentioned in the above-mentioned list for your convenience.

- Close the bottle's cap tightly so that no air can enter inside and mix all the mixtures well so that you can get the desired consistency out of it without any ambiguity on your way.

- Then keep the bottle in cool and dry place.

- Place the diffuser cap at the top of the bottle.

- Press the button to have its fumes out whenever you need.

Recipe no. 17

Ingredients:

- Almond essential oil 3 teaspoon

- Turmeric oil 3 drops

- Clementine oil 3 drops

- Clove bud oil 3 drops

Method:

- Take a small bottle or container and add all the ingredients that have been mentioned in the above-mentioned list for your convenience.

- Make the cap of the bottle closed and mix the oils well so that they can become smooth in consistency.

- Leave the bottle for about 3 days in a dry place or you can also place it in the sun for 3 to 3 hours daily so that the body spray can be enriched.

- Then keep the bottle at a place with the lowest level of humidity.

- Place the diffuser cap at the top of the bottle.

- Press the button to have its fumes out whenever you need.

Recipe no. 18

Ingredients:

- Rose essential oil 3 drops

- Rosemary essential oil 3 teaspoon

- Jasmine essential oil 3 teaspoon

- Apple cider vinegar half cup

Method:

- Take a small bottle or container and add all the ingredients that have been mentioned in the above-mentioned list for your convenience.

- Close the bottle's cap tightly so that no air can enter inside and mix all the mixtures well so that you can get the desired consistency out of it without any ambiguity on your way.

- Place the diffuser cap at the top of the bottle.

- Press the button to have its fumes out whenever you need.

Recipe no. 19

Ingredients:

- Coconut oil 3 teaspoon

- Rosemary essential oil 3 teaspoon

- Lemongrass oil 3 teaspoon

- Cumin oil 3 drops

- Vanilla oil 3 drops

- Sage oil 3 drops

Method:

- Take all the oils and ingredients.

- Take a small bottle or container and add all the ingredients that have been mentioned in the above-mentioned list for your convenience.

- Close the cap of the bottle and mix the oils well.

- Then keep the bottle in cool and dry place.

- Place the diffuser cap at the top of the bottle.

- Press the button to have its fumes out whenever you need.

Recipe no. 20

Ingredients:

- Rosemary oil 2 teaspoon

- Coconut oil 3 teaspoon

- Grapefruit oil 4 drops

- Celery seed oil 4 drops

- Black pepper oil 2 drops

Method:

- Take a small container and add all the ingredients that have been mentioned above.

- Beware that you are taking the right quantity just according to what have been mentioned in the ingredients above.

- Make the cap of the bottle closed and mix the oils well so that they can become smooth in consistency.

- Leave the bottle for about 3 days in a dry place or you can also place it in the sun for 3 to 3 hours daily so that the body spray can be enriched.

- Place the diffuser cap at the top of the bottle.

- Press the button to have its fumes out whenever you need.

Chapter 4 – 10 spring and summer essential oil diffuser recipes

Recipe no. 1

Ingredients:

Jojoba oil 4 drops

Almond oil 4 drops

Poppy seeds 2 teaspoon

Method:

- Mix all ingredients.
- Leave in dry place for about two days.
- Place the diffuser cap at the top of the bottle.
- Press the button to have its fumes out whenever you need.

Recipe no. 2

Ingredients:

Honey 4 drops

Jojoba oil 4 drops

Carrot oil 4 drops

Orange peel essential oil 2 drops

Method:

- Combine all ingredients.

- Leave in dry place for about two days.

- Place the diffuser cap at the top of the bottle.

- Press the button to have its fumes out whenever you need.

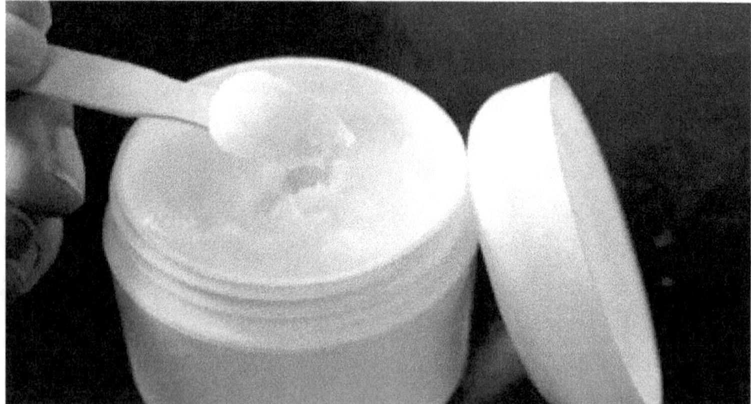

Recipe no. 3

Ingredients:

Jojoba oil 4 drops

Turmeric powder 1 teaspoon

Hazel drops 1 teaspoon

Method:

- Combine all ingredients.

- Then keep the bottle in cool and dry place.

- Place the diffuser cap at the top of the bottle.

- Press the button to have its fumes out whenever you need.

Recipe no. 4

Ingredients:

Lemon essential oil 4 drops

Almond oil 2 drops

Strawberry essential oil 2 drops

Method:

- Combine all ingredients.
- Then keep the bottle in cool and dry place.
- Place the diffuser cap at the top of the bottle.
- Press the button to have its fumes out whenever you need.

Recipe no. 5

Ingredients:

- Rose essential oil 3 drops

- Lemon oil 3 drops

Method:

- Take a small bottle or container and add all the ingredients that have been mentioned in the above-mentioned list for your convenience.

- Then keep the bottle in cool and dry place.

- Place the diffuser cap at the top of the bottle.

- Press the button to have its fumes out whenever you need.

Recipe no. 6

Ingredients:

Tea tree oil 2 teaspoon

Peppermint oil 1 teaspoon

Almond oil 4 drops

Method:

- Combine all ingredients.
- Then keep the bottle in cool and dry place.
- Place the diffuser cap at the top of the bottle.
- Press the button to have its fumes out whenever you need.

Recipe no. 7

Ingredients:

- Rose essential oil 3 drops

- Jasmine essential oil 3 drops

- Cumin oil 3 drops

- Lemon oil 3 drops

- Savory oil 3 drops

Method:

- Take a small bottle or container and add all the ingredients that have been mentioned in the above-mentioned list for your convenience.

- Close the bottle's cap tightly so that no air can enter inside and mix all the mixtures well so that you can get the desired consistency out of it without any ambiguity on your way.

- Then keep the bottle in cool and dry place.

- Place the diffuser cap at the top of the bottle.

- Press the button to have its fumes out whenever you need.

Recipe no. 8

Ingredients:

Jojoba oil 4 drops

Raspberry oil 2 teaspoon

Method:

- Combine all ingredients.

- Then keep the bottle in cool and dry place.

- Place the diffuser cap at the top of the bottle.

- Press the button to have its fumes out whenever you need.

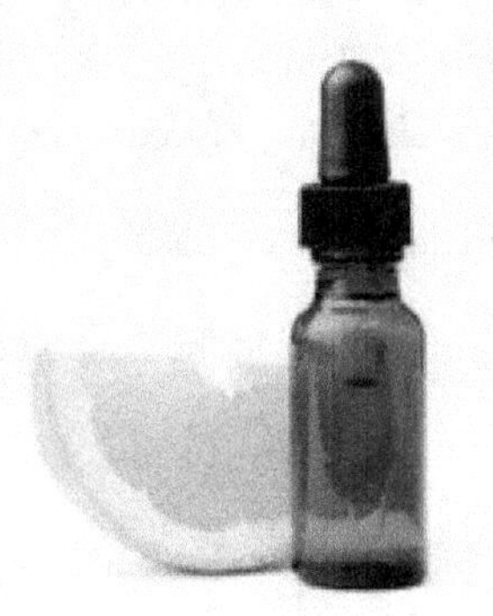

Recipe no. 9

Ingredients:

- Rose essential oil 3 drops

- Jasmine essential oil 3 drops

- Cumin oil 3 drops

- Lemon oil 3 drops

- Savory oil 3 drops

Method:

- Take a small bottle or container and add all the ingredients above.

- Close the bottle's cap tightly so that no air can enter inside and mix all the mixtures well so that you can get the desired consistency out of it without any ambiguity on your way.

- Then keep the bottle in cool and dry place.

- Place the diffuser cap at the top of the bottle.

- Press the button to have its fumes out whenever you need.

Recipe no. 10

Ingredients:

Jojoba oil 3 drops

Hazel 1 teaspoon

Almond oil 4 drops

Raspberry essential oil

Method:

- Combine all ingredients.

- Then keep the bottle in cool and dry place.

- Place the diffuser cap at the top of the bottle.

- Press the button to have its fumes out whenever you need.

Conclusion

The essential oils have got so many exceptional properties which can distinguish them from many other treatments as well. They sometimes act as anti-bacterial, anti-viral and antiseptic properties which are really helpful in getting out of all those problems which are caused by bacteria, virus or any other microbes.

Essential oils can grant you so many benefits which you cannot even imagine form any other source. Although, the modern people consider the use of modern medicines for curing many kinds of health problems but the use of essential oils is by far considered more effective and efficient as compared to any other thing. They can be used as summer diffusers and you will then not need to buy any deodorant from market again without any problem.

Organic Deodorant and Body Spray Recipes

Introduction

I want to thank you and congratulate you for downloading the book "Homemade Deodorant: 30 Best Non-Toxic Organic Deodorant and Body Spray Recipes to Keep You Dry And Smelling Fresh All Day Long!"

This book contains proven steps and strategies on how to make your own deodorant, body sprays, and perfumes.

The fact is commercial deodorants are not what they used to be. They are full of chemicals, harmful additives, and dyes that have been proven to be carcinogens, meaning they can cause cancer. In addition, they are endocrine disruptors, so they make you more susceptible to hormone abnormalities, which can also lead to cancer.

The bottom line is that deodorant that you purchase from the store is not healthy for you, but you can make your own version that works just as well, and doesn't come with the added risk of breast cancer, liver disease, and many other terrible complications!

Find out how to make your own deodorant, body spray, and perfume throughout this book.

Chapter One – Why Use Organic Ingredients?

Deodorant is a habitual practice that just about no one actually thinks about. It's a convenient roll on liquid, spray or a traditional stick application. Its purpose is to make sure that when you lift up your arms, no one has the pleasant surprise of smelling something unpleasant. Deodorant is your defense against wet underarms and smelly armpits, but what's in the current deodorant you might be wearing?

In this chapter, we're going to go over some of the common ingredients found in the conventional deodorant you might be purchasing, and see if these odor and sweat blocking additives are what you really want stuck to your underarms all day.

Once you understand the ingredients in conventional deodorant, you'll know why you should use organic ingredients to make your own deodorant.

Aluminum

Aluminum is the main ingredient that's included in antiperspirant deodorants. This is a metal that's used to block your sweat glands, decreasing your capability to sweat by an average of twenty percent. The problem with this common metal is that it can cause serious health risks such as breast cancer and Alzheimer's disease.

Due to aluminum's main function being to block the sweat glands, what happens to all of your sweat? The underarms are closely linked to the lymph nodes, so this accumulation of toxins from your sweat not being perspired can potentially cause mayhem in your armpits. No amount of build-up of toxins in your body is good for you, and long-term build-up can cause cell mutation.

While the link between aluminum and breast cancer has controversial studies, it still convincing them with most breast cancer is developing in the upper outer quadrant of the breasts, which is the close a squadron to your armpit with lymph nodes are located, the long-term use of commercial deodorant with aluminum is factored into the formation of certain breast cancers.

In addition, women are more likely to shave under their arms, which mean excess aluminum is able to pass through this area more effectively. This could be the reason why breast cancer is more common amongst women.

Propylene Glycol

Another ingredient that's frequently used in deodorants is propylene glycol. Propylene glycol is a substance that is derived from petroleum and use to make a soft and silky consistency. It's a cheap ingredient that has a versatile function, and this is the reason it's so common in beauty products. Propylene glycol acts as a penetration enhancer, so if it's paired with harmful chemicals it will increase their absorption.

Recent studies have shown that propylene glycol is considered to be nontoxic to the body when it's ingested. It's eliminated from the body after a few hours, which is why it's considered nontoxic. However, there are reports of its potential toxicity being linked to issues such as:

Cancer

Developmental abnormalities

Reproductive complications

Endocrine complications

Neurotoxicity

Propylene glycol has a single main concern beings that it's a skin sensitizer, which means it can cause allergic reactions such as irritant contact dermatitis, non-immunologic contact urticarial (hives), and allergic contact dermatitis.

Itching profusely under the arms can be very annoying, not to mention embarrassing.

Phthalates

This ingredient, also known as fragrance on the ingredient list, is a plasticizing chemical that's often used in many other beauty products due to their consistency and their capability to help dissolve some of the other ingredients.

The performance and the function of the ingredient seem to be more important to the conventional skin care brands than the quality and the safety of the ingredients.

This product helps your deodorant glide on smoothly, but what are the consequences of it being in your deodorant? It is worth having a temporary fix that could possibly cause a larger problem later on?

Phthalates are linked to many health issues and are considered endocrine disruptors. Once they are absorbed by your body, they act like estrogen, which not only conflict with hormonal function, but they also cause many other complications, such as:

Decreased sperm count

Infertility

Prostate, breast, and ovarian cancer

Lung, liver, and kidney damage

Asthma

Endometriosis

Allergies

These are a probable human carcinogen and while the United States continues to regulate them, they're still very prevalent in many beauty products, including deodorants.

Sometimes, you might not consider the potential harm of a simple step of getting ready in the morning, but little do you know that your deodorant, antiperspirants, and your body sprays are all just another pitfall in an endless chemical burden of the conventional skin care products.

So skip the dangerous commercial deodorants, body sprays, perfumes, and mists, and try out some of the recipes in this book!

Chapter Two – Organic Deodorant Recipes

Homemade Deodorant with Shea Butter

Ingredients

3 Tbsp. Coconut Oil

2 Tbsp. Shea Butter

3 Tbsp. Baking Soda

2 Tbsp. Arrowroot Powder

Essential Oils Of Your Choice

Directions

Melt the coconut oil and the Shea butter in a double boiler over medium heat until they're just melted. You want to combine in a quart sized glass mason jar with a lid instead and put this in a small saucepan of water until it's melted. This saves you a bowl and you can just designate this jar for this type of project and not need to wash it out. This can also be done in your microwave.

Remove this from the heat and add the arrowroot and the baking soda.

Mix it all together well.

Add the essential oils and then pour it all into a glass container to store it. It doesn't need to be refrigerated.

If you like, you can allow it to cool totally and put it into an old deodorant stick for easier usage, thought it could melt in the summer.

Take note this recipe can take a few hours to completely harden and the process can be sped up by putting it in the refrigerator for a few minutes.

Coconut Oil Homemade Deodorant Recipe

Ingredients

6 Tbsp. Coconut Oil

¼ C. Baking Soda

¼ C. Arrowroot Powder

Essential Oils Of Your Choice

Directions

Mix the arrowroot powder and the baking soda together in a medium bowl.

Mash the oil with a fork until it's well incorporated.

Add the oils if you prefer them.

Store it in a small, glass jar or an old deodorant container.

Deodorant Bar Recipe

Ingredients

½ C. Coconut Oil

½ C. Shea Butter

½ C. Beeswax

1 Tsp. Vitamin E Oil

3 Tbsp. Baking Soda

½ C. Organic Arrowroot Powder

3 Capsules High Quality Probiotics

20 Drops Essential Oil Of Your Choice

Directions

Combine the coconut oil, shea butter and the beeswax in a double boiler or a glass bowl that's set over a smaller saucepan with an inch of water in it. You can also use a quart sized glass mason jar with a lid and put it in a small saucepan of hot water. This saves you the bowl and you can designate the jar for this type of project and not have to wash it out.

Turn the burner on and bring your water to a boil. Stir the ingredients continuously until they're melted and smooth.

Remove them from the heat and add the vitamin E oil, arrowroot powder, baking soda, probiotics, and the essential oils. Be sure the oil isn't too hot so the heat won't kill your probiotics. If you can touch it without being burnt, it's not too hot.

Gently stir it until all the ingredients are well combined.

If you want to make this into bars, then pour it into muffin tins or another mold that will hold liquid. If you are going to put it into an old deodorant container and use it like stick deodorant, then let the mix harden for around twenty minutes. When it's around the consistency of peanut butter, use a spoon to scoop it into the tube and pack it down in. Then, allow the cup to stay off overnight to completely harden the deodorant before using it.

Homemade Deodorant for Sensitive Skin

Ingredients

¾ C. Cornstarch or Arrowroot Powder

¼ C. Baking Soda

6 Tbsp. Melted Coconut Oil

Directions

Combine the arrowroot powder or cornstarch with the baking soda.

Add four tablespoons of the coconut oil to the mix and mash it down with a fork until it's well combined. Keep adding the coconut oil until the deodorant reaches a consistency you like.

Transfer the mix to a jar that has a tight fitting lid.

To use the deodorant, apply a little under your arms with your fingertips as it's needed.

Homemade Deodorant Recipe for Sensitive Skin

Ingredients

¾ C. Cornstarch or Arrowroot Powder

¼ C. Diatomaceous Earth (Food Grade)

9 Tbsp. Melted Coconut Oil

Directions

Combine the arrowroot or cornstarch with the diatomaceous earth.

Add six tablespoons of melted oil and mix it up with a fork. Keep adding the oil until the deodorant has reached your desired consistency.

Then transfer to a jar that has a tight fitting lid and apply a small amount under your arms when it's needed.

All-Natural Homemade Deodorant Recipe

Ingredients

½ Tbsp. Baking Soda

⅛ C. Arrowroot Powder

⅛ C. Cocoa Butter

⅛ C. Shea Butter

5 Vitamin E Oil Drops

25-40 Drops Your Chosen Essential Oil

Directions

Using a Pyrex measuring glass, combine the shea butter and the cocoa butter.

Use a double boiler to heat the oils over medium heat until they are melted.

Remove them from the heat and stir in the baking soda and the arrowroot powder.

Stir in the vitamin E oil and your essential oils.

Carefully pour this mix into two ounce tins, filling them to the top, but making sure not to spill it over.

Put the lids on the container but don't press down to lock them. Just allow them to rest on the top to help prevent any dust from settling into the deodorant as it settles.

Let it completely cool and solidify, which can take six or more hours. Letting it sit overnight is best.

Homemade Deodorant

Ingredients

½ C. Coconut Oil

½ C. Baking Soda

40-60 Essential Oil Drops

Empty Deodorant Container

Directions

Put the oil into a bowl.

Mix the baking soda into it.

Add the essential oil and mix well.

Store it in your deodorant container or in a glass jar.

Recipe for Homemade Summer Deodorant

Ingredients

¼ C. Cornstarch

¼ C. Baking Soda

3 Tbsp. coconut Oil

1 Tbsp. Beeswax, Grated

5 Tea Tree Oil Drops

5 Essential Oil Drops of Your choice

Directions

Start by melting the oil and the wax together in a double boiler. Rest a heat-proof bowl inside a saucepan that has an inch worth of water in the bottom. Heat it gently, stirring continuously, until the wax has melted.

Add the rest of the ingredients.

Stir it together. At this point, you will have a runny paste or slurry. This changes quickly.

Work quickly by pouring the paste into the empty deodorant container. By the end of this step, you might have to scrape the last bit of paste into the container and push it down, smoothing the top. That's how quickly it will begin to solidify.

Lemon Juice

Ingredients

Lemon Juice

Directions

Many people like to use lemon as a natural deodorizer. Lemon juice contains citric acid that helps kill the odor-causing bacteria under your arms. Use a lemon slice on your armpits every morning. Remember, don't use lemon juice on any recently shaved areas, though!

Rubbing Alcohol

Ingredients

Rubbing Alcohol
Cotton Ball

Directions

Rubbing alcohol is another way to kill odor causing bacteria. It's inexpensive and very easy to use, too. You can just fill a spray bottle with rubbing alcohol and spritz it under your arms, or you can use a cotton ball and gently dab it on. Adding an essential oil will make it into a pretty, scented spritzer, too.

Detoxifying Deodorant

Ingredients

5 Tbsp. Coconut Oil

3 Tbsp. Baking Soda

3 Tbsp. Arrowroot Powder

2 Tbsp. Bentonite Clay

20 Tea Tree Oil Drops

Directions

Put everything in a mixing bowl in the order that it's listed in. because coconut oil is a solid when it's at room temperature, it has to be heated to be able to mix it easily. With your clean hands, knead the mixture until everything makes a smooth paste. Then transfer this paste to a glass jar or a deodorant stick.

The paste will thicken after you let it cool at room temperature. To apply it, just rub your finger on the top of the paste and scoop out a little amount to rub on your underarms. The pate will melt right into the sick and absorb quickly.

All-Natural Coconut Deodorant

Ingredients

¼ C. Coconut Oil

⅛ C. Cornstarch

⅛ C. Arrowroot Powder

Essential Oils of Your Choice

1 Tbsp. Baking Soda

Directions

Combine the oil, cornstarch, baking soda, and the arrowroot powder in a mixing bowl. When it's well combined, add in your essential oil a few drops at a time until you get to the scent you prefer.

Pour it into an empty deodorant container or just pour it into a small mason jar and refrigerator it for fifteen minutes. Remove it from the refrigerator and use it as you need it.

If you're using a mason jar, you'll need to chip out some little piece and then rub it onto your armpit. The deodorant melts and applies smoothly to your skin.

DIY Natural Deodorant Solid Recipe

Ingredients

2 Tbsp. Coconut Oil

1 Tbsp. Beeswax

1 Tbsp. Shea Butter

2 Tbsp. Arrowroot Powder

1 ½ Tbsp. Bentonite Clay

1 Tbsp. Baking Soda

2 Drops Citronella Essential Oil

2 Drops Lemongrass Essential Oil

2 Drops Tea Tree Essential Oil

Directions

In a double boiler, add the shea butter, coconut oil, and the wax. Bring it all to a boil over medium heat and stir until the wax and oils are melted.

Remove it from the heat and add in the bentonite clay, baking soda, arrowroot powder, and the essential oils. Mix it all well.

Pour the liquid into some silicone muffin molds or a five ounce container, such as an empty deodorant container.

Let it cool down and solidify for around two to three hours. The wax will help keep it solid so you can use it as a traditional deodorant.

Easy Deodorant

Ingredients

¼ C. Baking Soda

¼ C. Cornstarch or Arrowroot Powder

5 Tbsp. Coconut Oil

Directions

Combine the arrowroot powder and the baking soda together with a fork. Start with around four tablespoons of the oil and then add it to the baking soda mix. Work it into a paste.

Add the rest if you feel you need to.

You can store this in a small container or put it in an empty deodorant stick.

Vitamin E Deodorant

Ingredients

3 Tbsp. Shea Butter

2 Tbsp. Cornstarch

3 Tbsp. Baking Soda

2 Tbsp. Cocoa Butter

2 Vitamin E Caps

Essential Oil of your choice

Directions

Melt everything but the oil together and stir it.

The mix in the oil and pour it into a container, and put the container in the refrigerator to let it set.

This recipe will fill a ¼ pint jar.

Chapter Three – Organic Body Spray Recipes

Vanilla and Ylang-Ylang Body Spray

Ingredients

18 Vanilla Oleoresin Drops

2 Ylang-Ylang Drops

¼ C. Witch Hazel with Alcohol

Directions

Mix everything together in a dark colored spray bottle and store it in a dark place.

Vanilla and Sweet Orange Body Spray

Ingredients

16 Vanilla Oleoresin Drops

4 Sweet Orange Essential Oil Drops

¼ C. Witch Hazel with Alcohol

Directions

Mix everything together in a dark colored bottle and store it in a dark place.

Vanilla and Coffee Body Spray

16 Vanilla Oleoresin Drops

4 Coffee Essential Oil Drops

¼ C. Witch Hazel with Alcohol

Directions

Mix everything together in a dark colored spray bottle and store it in a dark, cool place.

Vanilla Clove Body Oil Spray

Ingredients

¼ C. Almond Oil

½ tsp. Vanilla Extract or Essential Oil

3 Drops Clove Oil

Spray Bottle

Directions

Combine the ingredients and pour it into a small spray bottle.

Orange Blossom Body Spray

Ingredients

1 oz. Filtered Water

90 Drops Orange Essential Oil

½ tsp. Vegetable Glycerine

Directions

Add everything to a small spray bottle, shake to combine and spritz onto your skin. Be sure to rub it in.

Bohemian Patchouli Body Spray

Ingredients

1 oz. filtered water

⅛ tsp. Tunisian Patchouli Essential Oil

½ tsp. Vegetable Glycerine

Directions

Mix it together in a small, glass spray bottle and shake it well. Shake it before you use it.

Citrus Energy Natural Body Spray

Ingredients

1 oz. Distilled Water

½ oz. Witch Hazel with Alcohol

½ oz. Vegetable Glycerin

10 Grapefruit Essential Oil Drops

4 Lime Essential Oil Drops

4 Lemon Essential Oil Drops

Directions

Mix everything together in a small glass bottle and shake it well. Shake it before every use.

Orange Vanilla Natural Body Spray

Ingredients

1 oz. Distilled Water

½ oz. Witch Hazel with Alcohol

½ oz. Vegetable Glycerin

⅛ tsp. Vanilla Extract

10 Drops Orange Essential Oil

Directions

Mix it all together in a small glass bottle and shake it well. Shake it before every use.

Purifying Linen and Body Spray

Ingredients

1 C. Water

120 Drops Essential Oil

20 Drops Peppermint

40 Drops Lemon

40 Drops Eucalyptus

Dark Brown Spray Bottle (Glass)

Directions

Pour the water into the bottle

Add the essential oils.

Shake before you use it.

Moisturizing Body Spray

Ingredients

¼ C. Distilled Water

1 ½ tsp. Vegetable Glycerin

1 tsp. Grapeseed Oil

5 Drops Vitamin E Oil

10 Drops Essential Oil

Directions

Combine all the ingredients and carefully pour them into a small spray bottle, around three ounces. Shake it well before you use it.

Spray it liberally on your body as it's needed, especially after you shower. Rub it into your skin.

Lemon, Lavender, and Vanilla Body Spray

Ingredients

1 Glass Spray Bottle, 4 oz.

3 ½ oz. Vodka

5 Drops Lemon essential Oil

15 Drops Lavender Essential Oil

30 Drops Vanilla Essential Oil

Directions

Combine everything into a spray bottle and shake it well before using it.

Woodland Body Spray

Ingredients

4 Drops Spruce Essential Oil

2 Drops Cedarwood Essential Oil

2 Drops Fir Needle Essential Oil

1 Drop Bergamot Essential Oil

1 Drop Vetiver Essential Oil

1 tsp. Jojoba Oil

Directions

Add all the essential oils into the glass bottle and mix the oils with a wooden skewer or by shaking it gently.

Add the oil and shake it again.

Add more essential oil if you want it to be a little stronger.

Cucumber, Aloe Body Mist

Ingredients

1 Squeeze Lemon

1 Cucumber

1 tsp. Aloe Vera Gel

1 Tbsp. Rosewater

Directions

Peel the cucumber and dice it into pieces. Put them in a blender and pulse it on high for around a minute.

Cover a bowl with some cheese cloth and then strain the juice into the bowl.

Add the rest of the ingredients to the bowl and mix it thoroughly.

Transfer the mix to a spray bottle and you're done. You can add a little distilled water if you feel you need to dilute it a bit.

Store it in the refrigerator so it doesn't spoil. It'll last around a week.

Tropical Body Mist

Ingredients

1 oz. Distilled Water

10ml Rose Hydrosol

2 tsp. Vanilla Extract

1 tsp. Vodka

1 Tbsp. Vegetable Glycerin

1 Tbsp. Coconut Oil

5 Grapefruit Essential Oil drops

15 Neroli Essential Oil Drops

Directions

Begin by filling the spray bottle with some lukewarm distilled water and the hydrosol.

Add the vegetable glycerin slowly and then add the coconut oil. Use a wooden skewer to mix the two.

Make sure you're happy with the scent thus far and the consistency.

Then add the essential oils and close the spray bottle. Shake it well.

Let it rest a few hours before you use it the first time.

Always shake it well to make sure all the ingredients are mixed well.

Vanilla Cardamom Mist

Ingredients

6 Cardamom Seeds

½ C. Water

1 tsp. Vanilla Extract

Directions

Crack the seeds to expose their pods.

Put the bits of cardamom into a saucepan with the water and bring it to a boil. Remove it from the heat.

Let the cardamom water cool totally.

Transfer the scented water to a spray bottle.

Add the vanilla, seal the spray bottle, and shake it.

Adjust the amount of vanilla extract to your preference and store in a cool, dry place.

Grapefruit Mist

Ingredients

10 Drops Grapefruit Essential Oil

Vodka

Distilled Water

Glass Spray Bottle

Directions

Fill the glass bottle up around two-thirds of the way with the vodka and add a few drops of the essential oil before you fill the bottle up the rest of the way with the distilled water.

Chapter Four – Organic Perfume Recipes

Solid Perfume

Ingredients

1 ½ Tbsp. Beeswax

1 ½ Tbsp. Olive Oil

40 Drops Essential Oil of your choice

Directions

Fill up a pan with half a cup of water and put it on the burner. Turn the burner heat to medium. Put the wax beads into a heatproof glass bowl and put it inside the pan. When it's melted, mix in the oil. Let it melt for another five minutes.

Remove the glass owl from the pan and quickly stir in the essential oil. Pour this into its final container.

The essential oils will smell strong in the beginning, but they will fade over time.

To use the solid perfume, wipe it on the interior of your wrist for a clean scent that'll last all day.

California Citrus Sunshine

Ingredients

1 Tbsp. Jojoba Oil

2 Tbsp. Grain Alcohol

7 Drops Sweet Orange Essential Oil

7 Drops Grapefruit Essential Oil

7 Drops Peppermint Essential Oil

7 Drops Lavender Essential Oil

1 Tbsp. Distilled Water

Directions

Begin by adding the jojoba to a glass container and then add the alcohol. It's important to use glass and not plastic.

Add the essential oils in the order they were listed in on the ingredients list.

Add the distilled water using a dropper.

Mix the ingredient well and transfer them to a dark container for forty-eight hours up to six weeks. The longer it sits, the stronger the scent is going to be.

Transfer it to a pretty perfume bottle after it's reached your desired scent.

Solid Shimmer Perfume

Ingredients

2 tsp. almond oil

Essential oils of your choice

1 oz. beeswax

Directions

To make the solid perfume, combine the almond oil with the essential oils until you reach your desired scent.

The melt the wax and in a small glass in your microwave and add the oil mix. Stir it to combine it. Then pour it into a small mold to let it harden.

Add a small amount of shimmery eye shadow to give it some sparkle.

How to make Solid Essential Oil Perfume

Ingredients

1 Tbsp. beeswax

1 ½ Tbsp. Jojoba Oil

70 Drops Essential Oil

Directions

Grate or chop the beeswax finely and put it in the milk jug. Measure the oil into a small glass and then add the essential oil drops to your desired scent.

Melt the wax by filling the saucepan with about an inch of water, and then putting a glass container in the water. Put the beeswax into the glass and avoid spilling any water into the glass. Bring the water to a simmer and melt the wax.

As soon as it's done, add the oil and stir it with a wooden skewer until it's well combined. Carefully remove it from the hot water. The glass is going to be hot, so use a cloth to protect your hands.

Quickly pour the wax into containers and let it rest for half an hour or until it's cooled down. To use it, just rub the wax surface with your fingertips and then rub it on your wrists and neck.

Lavender Vanilla Mist

Ingredients

½ C. Vodka

2 Tbsp. Vegetable Glycerin

1 C. Dried Lavender Flowers

2 Vanilla Beans

10 Drops Vanilla Extract

15 Drops lavender Essential Oil

Directions

Slice the vanilla bean open with a sharp knife.

Put the beans and the flowers in a large glass jar with a lid.

Pour the vodka into the jar and secure the lid.

Let the mix infuse for a week.

Strain and discard your vanilla beans and your lavender flowers.

Add the lavender essential oil, the glycerin, and the vanilla extract to the reserved liquids and stir it well.

Replace the lid and let it age for four to six weeks.

Strain the perfume once again through a paper filter and then transfer it to a decorate spray bottle.

Midnight Perfume

Ingredients

2 Tbsp. Jojoba Oil or Grape Seed Oil

6 Tbsp. Vodka

2 ½ Tbsp. Distilled Spring Water

Funnel

Coffee Filter

Essential Oils

15 Drops Clove Oil

6 Drops Cedarwood Oil

9 Drops lavender Oil

2 Dark Colored Glass Bottles

Decorate Perfume Bottle

Directions

Start by cleaning the bottles, either in the dishwasher on the hottest setting or with some hot, soapy water. Put the bottles on a rimmed baking sheet and dry them in an oven set at 230 degrees Fahrenheit. Remove them from the oven when they're totally dry.

Put a lid on one of them and set it aside until you need it, which will anywhere from two days to six weeks later.

Put the carrier oil in one of your bottles.

Then add the essential oils.

Add the vodka.

Put the lid on top of the bottle and shake it well for several minutes.

Let it rest for forty-eight hours to six weeks.

The scent changes over time, becoming its strongest around six weeks.

Check it weekly and once you're happy with the scent, add two tablespoons of spring water to it and shake it well for a minute.

Put the coffee filter into the funnel and transfer your perfume from the bottle it's in to the perfume bottle. Label it and store it in a cool, dark place.

Citrus Lavender

Ingredients

2 tsp. Beeswax

48 Drops Essential Oils

12 Drops Sweet Orange Essential Oil

12 Drops Lemon Essential Oil

12 Drops lavender Essential Oil

12 Drops Bergamot Essential Oil

2 tsp. Jojoba Oil

½ oz. Tin

Directions

It's a good idea to blend the oils first before you begin working with the beeswax because it will harden very quickly.

Put all your essential oils into one cup so you can pour them into the beeswax mix when it's time.

You can play around with the amount of oil that you use and try to substitute different ones if you don't like the ones that were listed.

You can also use sweet almond oil for the carrier oil, too.

In another cup from the essential oils, measure out two teaspoons of the oil of your choice.

Measuring out the oil ahead of time saves you from having to rush around once the wax has melted.

If you have pellets of wax, then measure out two teaspoons of them into a small saucepan over medium to low heat.

If you have a block of wax, then you should grate off around a tablespoon of wax and then melt them in the pot. Then measure to make sure you have two teaspoons.

After you measure, you may find you have to heat the wax up again in the pan a few more seconds because it might begin to harden after you pour it into a measuring spoon.

Once you have the two teaspoons of the melted beeswax, add the carrier oil to it and stir it around until they're both combined.

Then take the pot off the burner and very quickly add the essential oils. Stir until they are well combined.

As quickly as you can, pour the mix into the container.

Cover it and allow it to rest ten minutes before you enjoy it.

Conclusion

Thank you again for downloading this book!

I hope this book was able to help you to learn how to make your own deodorant.

The next step is to gather up your ingredients and start cooking!

Finally, if you enjoyed this book, please take the time to share your thoughts and post a review on Amazon. It'd be greatly appreciated!

Thank you and good luck!

25 Best Homemade Soap Recipes for Home

Introduction

Research suggests that soap was being used as long ago as 2800 B.C. The ancient Babylonians are thought to have made soap from ashes and fat, although it is unknown as to the extent that soap was used by the general population.

There is also evidence to suggest that the Ancient Egyptians, from approximately 1500 B.C. used a soap product created by mixing fatty animal oils with salt; in effect create a soap which would exfoliate as well! Even the Romans are known to have made a form of soap from urine!

Soap is, in effect a vital part of human history, whether washing blood from your hands in ancient times or destroying microscopic germs; it has always been used. Of course, the more modern versions of soap have been created to leave a pleasant aroma as well as effective and gently washing the skin.

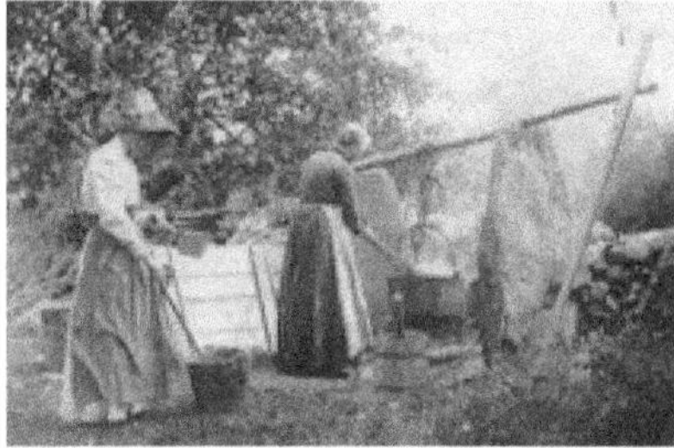

As with most products, soap was originally something that only the richest people could afford; there were very few people capable or licensed to make soap and they guarded their skills carefully. They general used animal oil and parts of plants to create distinctive soaps. This ensured an elite class of customer. However, at the end of the 18th century, a Frenchman discovered a way of chemical making soap; this was the first time soap could be made on a much larger scale. This was the catalyst which drove the price of soap down and made it affordable to a much wider range of people.

This discovery was followed in the early part of the 19th century that soap could be made from glycerin, fats and acid. This made it even cheaper to create soap and is considered to be the foundations of modern soap making; there have been no significant advancements in the science of soap making since. The techniques and principles which were first used approximately two hundred years ago, are still in use today!

Of course, modern technology has changed the understanding of soap, he ingredients are better understood and broken down which has enabled the creation of different types of soap for different situations. Laundry soap is one example of a product which is subtly different to hand soap or even bathing soaps; each has its own role to fulfill. It was only in the 1970's that liquid soap became possible, it has become exceptionally popular since and helps to promote hand washing as well as minimize soap wastage.

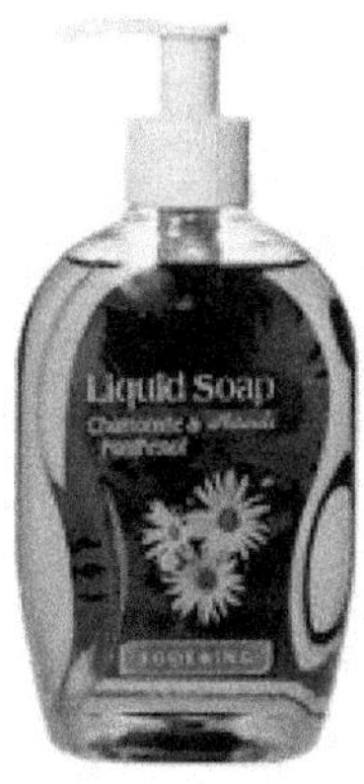

The modern world has a dazzling array if soaps, depending upon your needs, how you wish to smell and even what type of skin you have. These constant changes, improvements and marketing ploys help to keep soap fresh in everyone's mind; a standard bar of soap may be less popular, but the concept and use of soaps has never been so popular. There remains a thriving market for commercially created soaps, there is also a place for those who wish to create their own, homemade soap; a process which I surprisingly easy!

This book will guide you through the best method to make soap and the tools and equipment you will need to complete this task at home. It will also provide you with a selection of twenty five recipes to help you practice and create your own soap; you should then be able to discover and make hundreds of other types of soap!

Chapter 1 – The Need For Soap and How to Make It

In the modern world everyone is aware of the need for soap and its role in helping us to stay clean and healthy, although many people are unaware of how soap works and how regularly it should be used. In fact, there have been many studies into the effects of soap. There are even those who believe that soap is not necessary; the body is able to clean itself. There are two main uses of soap:

Odor Removal

In general research agrees that young children, male or female do not have any odor creating regions. It is, therefore, not necessary for children to use soap in order to remove unpleasant body odors, although soap can still be used to aid them in smelling nice. However, adults, particularly men, do have odor producing regions. Research suggests that it is essential to soap these regions every two days unless you partake in very physical work; in which case every day is essential. Water by itself can significantly reduce the presence if body odor, but will not eliminate it completely. Deodorant will always be needed to assist with reducing and containing odors, the regularity of application will be directly related to the physical duties undertaken. Washing in water will help to reduce body odor but it is more effective when mixed with soap.

Cleanliness

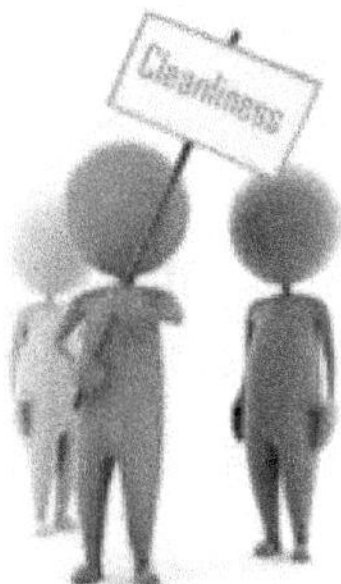

Soap has always been acknowledged as a way to remove dirt and germs from your hands, this is via a process of friction and agitation; in fact, modern soaps have small particles added to them to aid with dirt removal and the removal of excess skin. The abrasive nature of these products will help to leave your skin fresh and glowing and will often help to keep skin conditions at bay. This is because many soap products are becoming more technologically advanced and are able to offer deep pore washes.

There is a school of thought which recommends using only water to clean the skin. However, with the advancements in modern science washing soap can do much more than simple wash your skin, it can help t protect, moisturize and even keep you looking younger for longer.

It is the amount of science behind the soap that often worries people regarding what they are really putting on their face or body. This is one of the main reasons people start to make their own soap; knowing which ingredients have been placed into a bar means you know what you are putting on your body.

The basic process of making any soap is surprisingly simple, in fact, the most important question you will need to ask yourself is whether you wish to handle Lye yourself or not.   Lye is a natural product, also known as Sodium Hydroxide. It is an alkali and can be dangerous; it is capable of making a hole in your fabrics and can burn your skin. However, as long as you handle it with care there will be no issue using it; it is worth noting that you should always use the crystal version of Lye when making salt and it must always be added to the water, not the water to it.

This lye, added in the right quantities to plain water can then be mixed with a variety of different oil. The mixture bonds together to create soap; the main difference between recipes is the additional flavorings and the type of oil used. Every oil has its own specific relationship to lye and must be used in the right quantities.

If the thought of handling lye is to daunting for you at first, then you can purchase a melt and pour soap which is ready to use. As its name suggests, you simply melt it, add your own flavors and pour it into the molds.

The basic tools and equipment required are covered in the next chapter.

Chapter 2 – Tools and Equipment

Thankfully most of the items you will need you will already own; they are normal kitchen utensils. It is worth noting that if you intend to create your own soap on a regular basis is could be worth purchasing equipment specifically for your soap making. This will ensure there is no tang of soap left when cooking your evening meal!

Of course, as well as having all the right tools to hand, you will need to have chosen one of the recipes in this book and made sure that you either have the necessary ingredients or that you have acquired. It can be surprisingly cost effective, as well as fun to make your own soap.

Essential Tools;

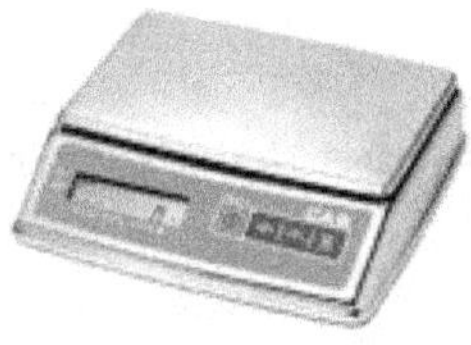

- Scales – the best ones are digital as the more soap you make the more precise you will be regarding the ingredients. This is not just in an effort to reproduce a bar of soap; very small changes in the ingredients can affect the oiliness of the finished product.

- Jars and bowls; these should, ideally, be made of glass.

- Spoons; the best option is to have a wooden one, a metal one and a plastic one.

- Something to contain and shape your soap. You can buy purpose made molds, or you can use a variety of items from your home. Silicon cake tins are one option, but a cardboard box lined with parchment paper can work just as well.

- Gloves are essential as the mixture will be hot, if you decide to use Lye it can also be harmful to your skin. It is also advisable to have some sort of eye protection; this will help prevent splashes from damaging your eyes.

- Vinegar – this will effectively counteract the lye if you do have an accident with it. Having a bottle to hand means you will be ready and able to prevent a disaster!

- A blender; this will make mixing and creating your soap much easier! This should be the handheld, stick type.

- A mixing bowl; the size of this will depend upon the amount of soap you wish to make. For your first attempts it is advisable to make a small amount and get a feel for how to make soap; you will then be able to tweak recipes to suit your own requirements.

- Cloths; you will need to react quickly to any spills; a cloth or paper towel is the best option for this.

You may also wish to consider having a selection of plastic cups handy; this will help you to have the oils and fragrances pre-measured and ready to add to your mix.

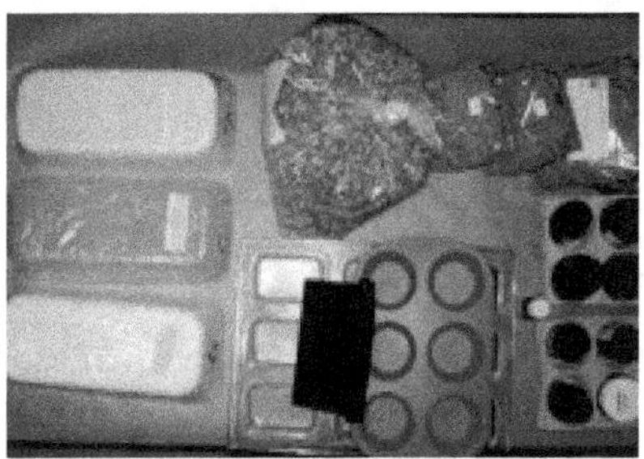

Having got all your tools to hand and your ingredients you will be ready to get started. Perhaps the most important thing to remember when making soap is that preparation is everything. You variety of containers will ensure you are able to measure and prepare all the ingredients before you start mixing them together; doing this will make the process much easier.

Chapter 3 – 10 Fantastic Soaps for All Occasions

There are literally hundreds of potential combinations and types of soap which can be made. In fact, some if the best ones are made as a result of trial and error. The best approach to learning how to make soap is to use the recipes in this book, follow the instructions and understand the process. Once you have mastered this you will be able to change the ingredients and try some of your own combinations, just be sure to note down what you are doing so that you can reproduce it if necessary!

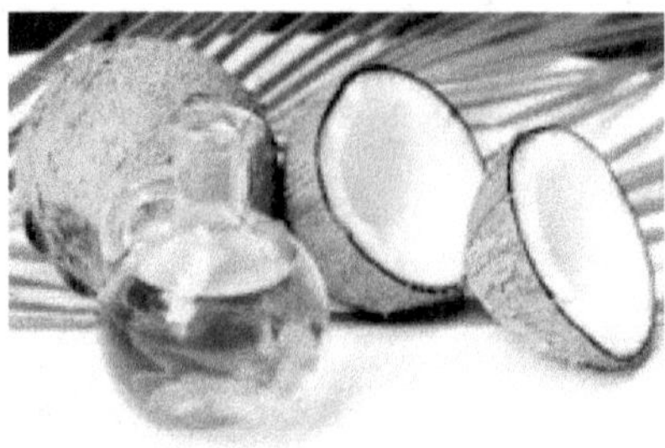

Coconut Oil Soap for Washing

You will need 33 ounces of Coconut Oil, 4.75 ounces of lye and 12.5 ounces of water. If you wish to you can also an a few drops of essential oils.

It is worth noting that there are various types of coconut oil which melt at different temperatures. Ideally you should use one which melts at 76 degrees Fahrenheit, although the recipe will work well with any coconut oil.

The first step is to measure out your three key ingredients. You need to add the water to an empty bowl and then slowly pour the lye into the water. It is advisable to avoid breathing in the fumes whilst doing this. By pouring the lye slowly you will reduced the chance of splash-back and help it to dissolve effectively. The mixture will take approximately ten minutes to go clear.

Separately you will need to put your coconut oil into a pan and heat it to around 120 Fahrenheit. It should melt into a clear liquid.

You can then merge the two liquids carefully together. You can then use your blender to gentle mix it until it appears creamy and light. You can then put the mixture on a low heat and allow to simmer for approximately three quarters of an hour. The soap should be half clear; much like Vaseline. You can check it is ready by making sure it is between seven and ten on a piece of PH paper.

As it cools add your essential oils and then spoon the mixture into your chosen molds. It can cool naturally or cool in the fridge for a quicker result. It is usable straight away although it will be at its best a couple of weeks after production.

Coconut Oil Laundry Soap

This is the same ingredients as the soap for washing but it is important to use one ounce more of lye and half an ounce less of water. The rest of the process is the same but it will make a bar which is more appropriate for washing clothes in.

Olive Oil Soap

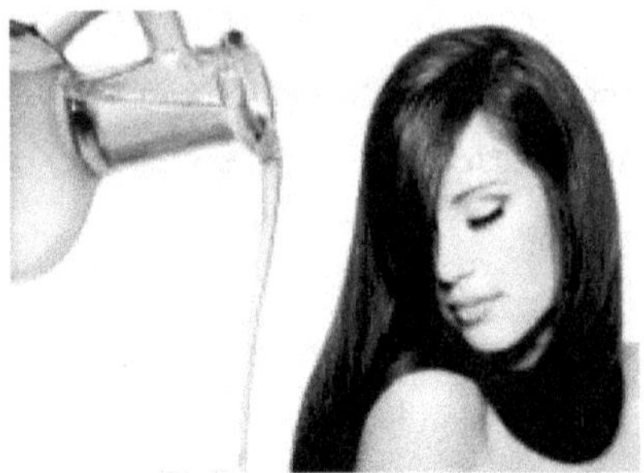

The ingredients in this are very similar to those in coconut oil soap. You will need 50 oz of olive oil, 6.3 oz of Lye and 15 oz of water.

You can choose whether to make the lye first or the olive oil. The water needs to be placed into a good sized bowl or container and the lye slowly added. Again, it will take approximately ten minutes to dissolve completely.

The olive oil will need heating on the stove to ensure it is hot, but not necessarily boiling. You can then slowly add this to the lye mixture and start blending. It should take between five and ten minutes to become nice and creamy.

You will then be able to fill your prepared molds and leave to set. They should, ideally be left overnight and they must be covered to ensure they harden properly.

Poppy seed Soap

Instead of using lye it is possible to use a soap base. This can be bought at most craft shops and will vary in price depending upon what the base is created from.

You will also need poppy seeds and you may wish to use coloring to ensure you soap look good.

Ideally you should use 10 oz of your soap base. Cut it into small pieces and place in a jug or bowl. This can then be melted in the microwave. Once melted add a teaspoon of poppy seeds and a few drops of coloring if required. You can also add a fragrance if desired. Mix all the ingredients and pour into your mold.

Put the mold in the fridge for fifteen minutes and then the soap is ready to us.

Jasmine and Rosewood

You will need one teaspoon of kaolin clay, two teaspoons of titanium dioxide, half an ounce of jasmine and half an ounce of rosewood. You will also need five ounces of lye, twelve ounce of water and possibly yellow oxide.

Start by adding the lye slowly to the water and leaving it to clear, (as before). Then mix the titanium dioxide and clay together; you will need to grind them to ensure there are no lumps. You can then add the jasmine, rosewood and titanium mixture to the lye, stirring carefully whilst doing so. You may also wish to add a little yellow oxide to improve the color of the soap.

Once mixed, you can pour into your chosen molds and leave for twenty four hours before cutting into blocks. It is best to leave the cut soap for three weeks before using it.

Calendula soap

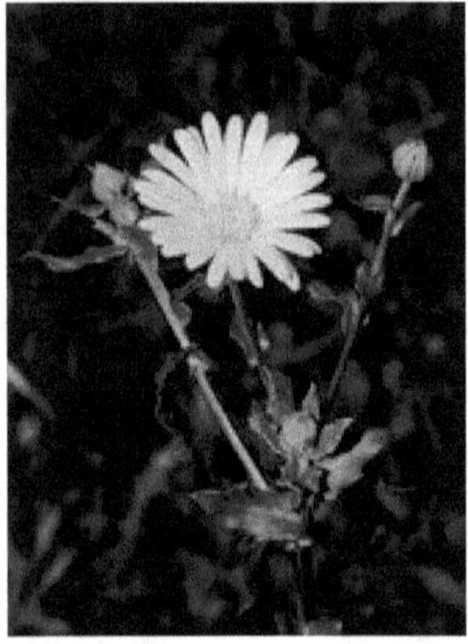

You will need; 21 ounces of olive oil, 14 ounces of coconut oil, 2 ounces of castor oil, 5 ounces of sunflower oil, 13 ounces of calendula tea, 6 ounces of lye and 13 ounces of water.

As usual measure out the water and slowly add the lye to it, then wait for it to become clear. Mix the oils together and heat them until they nearly reach boiling point, the slowly add them to the lye mix. Now simply add the calendula tea and blend until creamy.

You will then be able to pour them into your molds and use your soap in a couple of weeks.

Shampoo bar

As its name suggests this product is perfect for washing your hair! You will need; 9 ounces of olive oil and coconut oil, 4 ounces of coconut oil and of jojoba oil, two ounces of shea butter and cocoa butter, one ounce beeswax, four ounces water and four ounces of lye,

As usual, slowly add the lye to the water. Whilst this is becoming clear, mix all the oils and the beeswax together. This mixture can then be heated, but not brought to the boil. Now mix the lye with the oils and b lend until it is thick and creamy. The mixture should then be allowed to simmer for one hour and then you can pour it into its molds. After twenty four hours the mold can be cut into bar and left to cool further; although they can be used straight away.

Gin and Tonic Soap

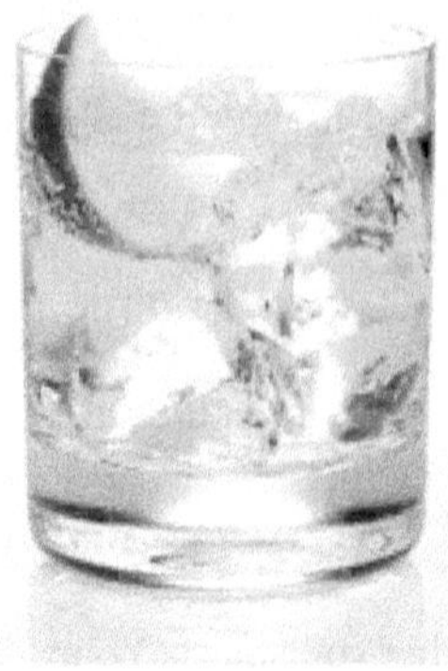

As with all the recipes you will need to pour 5 ounces of lye into 12 ounces of water and allow it to mix to makes its own, clear liquid.

You will then need to heat 3.5 ounces of olive oil, 2.5 ounces coconut oil, 1.5 ounces shea butter, 1.5 ounces lard and 1 ounce of castor oil. Do not allow it to boil before you add it the lye and water. This should then be left for approximately six hours; then add half an ounce of juniper oil, 3 ounces of lemon essential oil and a teaspoon of kaolin clay. Cut after twenty four hours and use after three weeks.

Lanolin Shaving soap

Lanolin is a natural moisturizer and is perfect for shaving with as it prevents the skin from drying out as you shave. To create it you will need the following ingredients:

1 ounce kokum butter, 2 ounces lanolin, 2 ounces of shea butter, 11 ounces of coconut oil, 10 ounces of rice bran oil, 7 ounces palm kernel flakes, 1 ounce

pumpkin oil. You will also need 5 ounces of lye and twelve ounces of water and you can add any essential oil you like to create a pleasant fragrance.

Mix the water and lye as usual, whilst waiting for it to cool and clear you should mix all the other oils and butter together, heat all these ingredients until they are all melted. Ideally you should merge the two liquids at approximately 110 degrees. Just prior to merging you can add the essential oils.

Once merged blend into a cream and then put into your molds. Keep them wrapped and insulated for twenty four hours before cutting them to size. Then keep them stored for another three weeks before using them.

Aloe Vera Soap

As with all these soaps you will need to prepare a mixture of lye and water before mixing the oils whilst heating and then combining the two mixtures. For this recipe you need 10 ounces of lye and 7 ounces of lye.

The oils which need to be mixed are 15 ounces Coconut oil, 13 Ounces olive oil and 10 ounces lard. Just prior to mixing them with the lye, it is essential to add the aloe gel. Once they have been blended it will take about 48 hours for them to be set enough to cut and a further four weeks before they should be used.

Chapter 4 – 10 Food Flavoured Soap

There are a great many number of soaps which have been created using food flavorings; this can add a beautiful fragrance to any soap and can also provide a host of health benefits. The following recipes all use the same approach as the soaps already described. Every soap mixture requires 12 ounces of water and 5 ounces of lye. Your soap making should start by carefully mixing these together. The mixture will go cloudy and become extremely hot. Whilst this is settling you should mix the oils and warm them. Add any essential oils can be added prior to mixing lye and the oils.

The following recipes all adopt this approach, as such, only the ingredients and items which need to be noted will appear:

Honey Soap

Additional ingredients to the lye and water are; one tablespoon of buttermilk fragrance oil, half a tablespoon of vanilla flavoring, orange color, (you can choose not to use this) and 3 ounces of honey. Your choice of honey will affect the color of your soap and hence affect whether you wish to use the orange coloring or not. You may also like to find bee molds or honeycombs to make the soap more fun!

Chai Latte Soap

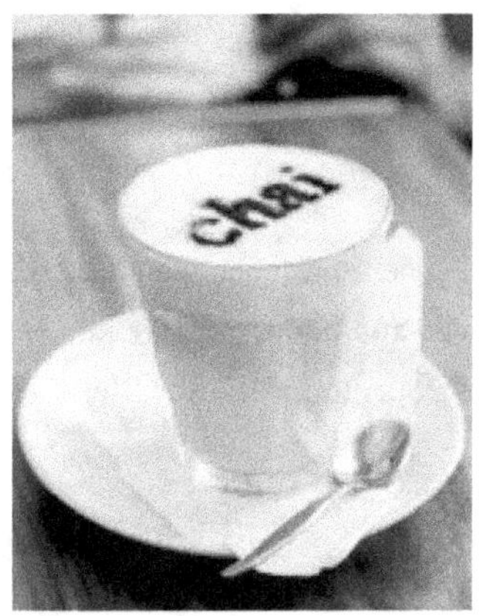

You will need five ounces of coconut oil, five ounces of olive oil and five ounces of olive oil. You will then also need two ounces of cocoa butter and two ounces of castor oil. The ingredients should all be mixed and blended as per the usual instructions. However, you will notice it thickens quickly when blended. It can also look fantastic to make them in plastic cups; you can even decorate the top and make two batches to create the milky layer and the coffee layer; so that they look like a coffee/ latte!

Chocolate Soap

Who wouldn't want to wash in a bar of chocolate! This soap is created to look exactly like a bar of chocolate, or, if stood on its end it could be a hot chocolate!

You will need; four ounces of olive oil, two and a half ounces of coconut oil, two ounces of lard, one ounce of avocado oil and half an ounce of castor oil. You will also need two teaspoons of whole milk powder, two of coffee granules, one teaspoon of cocoa powder and 2 teaspoons of vanilla flecks.

Additionally, you will need two teaspoons of red clay and two of brown clay, along with two teaspoons of vanilla flavoring.

The oils should be mixed with the lye as usual; once it has been blended and become creamy you can add the extra ingredients and pour into a mold. As usual the soap can be cut to size within twenty four hours and then left for three weeks to harden

Candy cane Christmas Soap

You will need; 4 ounces of olive oil, 2.5 ounces of coconut oil, 2 ounces of lard, 1 ounce of avocado oil and half an ounce of castor oil. You will also need two teaspoons of peppermint essence, one teaspoon of vanilla essence, one tablespoon kaolin clay, half a teaspoon of red oxide and half a teaspoon of green oxide.

Mix the lye and heat the oils as normal. Then add the vanilla and peppermint essence and blend in the kaolin clay. Now split the soap mix into three bowls. Add the red oxide to one bowl and the green oxide to another. Now alternate and swirl the colors separately into the molds. They should create a candy cane effect. As usual leave for twenty four hours before cutting and leave for a further thre weeks before using.

Milk Soap

You will need 20 ounces of milk, twenty ounces of coconut oil, four ounces of your preferred fragrance and four pounds of lard. As usual you can start by preparing the lye and water. You will need to wait for approximately an hour for the mixture to lower its temperature to approximately eighty degrees. You can then add the cold milk. Whilst the temperature is settling again you can prepare the oil and the lard; merging them and heating them to ninety degrees. You can then add the oils to the lye and keep stirring until it is thick.

You can then pour it into your chosen molds, but you must cover the mold with plastic and a blanket; this will ensure the heat is retained which will effectively cook the soap. Again, after twenty four hours it can be cut into shapes or the size required. It should be allowed to air dry for another four weeks before being used.

Creamy Orange Soap

This soap requires two tablespoons of annatto seeds, two ounces of olive oil, two tablespoons of poppy seeds, one ounce of essential oil; orange flavored preferably and one and a half ounces of peppermint oil.

Mix the oils heat them with the essential oils and seeds. The simply merge them with the lye mixture and blend. You should then be able to pour the mixture into the mold and leave for twenty four hours to set.

The seeds will act as an exfoliate in the soap making it very good at restoring dry skin.

Marbled Beer Soap

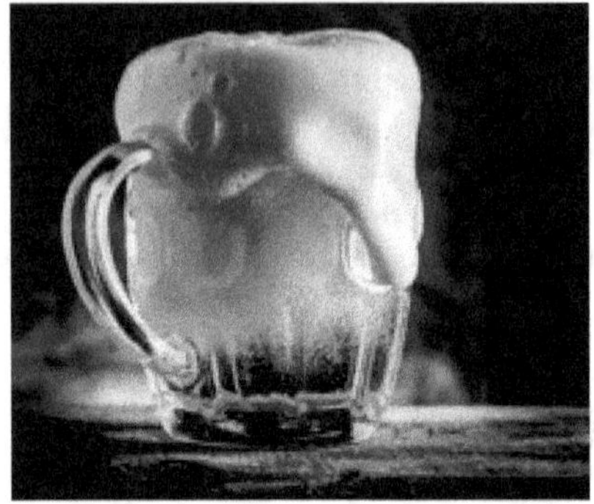

You may not know whether to wash with this or drink it, but it will certainly make a good talking point and a gift. You need four and a half ounces of chilled beer, five ounces of palm kernel oil, three and a half ounces of palm oil and the same of coconut oil. You will also need one ounce of Babassu oil, five ounces of rapeseed oil, five ounces of sunflower oil, one ounce of castor oil, two ounces of soybean oil and half an ounce of cedar wood essential oil.

Having collected all the ingredients together you should introduce half of the lye to the water as normal; the other half should be poured into the cold beer.

Heat your oils and merge them with your water and with your beer; roughly half the oils inn each pot. You will not be able to blend this to a thick consistency. Now pour the two mixtures into the mold, you can alternate or even pour at the same time to achieve a marble effect. You can then cover it for between twenty four and forty eight hours, keeping it warm to help it set.

Apple Cider Soap

In this mixture, instead of adding your lye to water, add it to nine ounces of chilled cider. You can then mix your oils; 15 ounces of olive oil, 2 ounces castor oil, 8 ounces coconut oil, 2 ounces cocoa butter and 3 ounces of avocado oil. You can also add a touch of ginger or cinnamon, to your own preference.

Cinnamon Soap

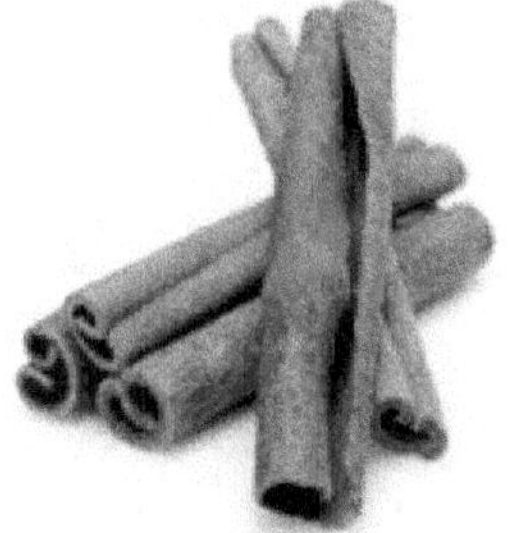

The oil mixture consists of 3.5 ounces olive oil, 2.5 ounces coconut oil, 1.5 ounces lard, 1.5 ounces shea butter and 1 ounce castor oil. You will also need a teaspoon of ground cinnamon, a tablespoon of white clay and two teaspoons of cinnamon essential oil. The essential oil, ground cinnamon and clay should

be added at the end of the process; just before you pour the soap into the
molds.

Tea Tree Soap

This soap requires an oil mixture of 14 ounces olive oil, 10 ounces coconut oil,
4 ounces sweet almond oil, 4 ounces avocado oil and two teaspoons of tea tree
essential oil. Again, the tea tree essential oil should be added just before the
soap is poured into the mold. After twenty four hours you can cut the mold
and it can be left to air dry for up to six weeks.

Chapter 5 – A selection of fun Soaps – 5 Recipes

The list of soaps you can make is endless; in fact, you are only limited by your imagination. It is even possible to use a soap base instead of the lye to avoid the danger involved in dealing with lye. The following five recipes are done using a soap base but are all worth trying: Each recipe requires you to melt the soap base in the microwave and then add the necessary ingredients to make your soap. Solid particles will go to the bottom of the soap unless you allow it to set a little first. The soap can set in as little as three hours although it is always recommended to chill it overnight.

Herbs & Citrus Soap

Simply put some soap base in a bowl, or grate an old bar of soap and warm it up. Soap base can be warmed in the microwave whereas old soap is best to do on the stove. Simply choose your favorite hers, such as mint or rosemary and grind or puree them into tiny pieces. Once your base has melted, and them to it and stir in. Pour the soap into the molds and leave to cool for an hour; you can speed the cooling and setting process by putting them in the freezer.

Mocha Soap

Simply melt the soap base and add approximately one tablespoon of coffee and cocoa powder to it. This will create a fantastic smelling soap. To help create the mocha effect you could melt a second soap base and add a little white colorant to help create the milky mocha effect. To make a stunning display pour the two soap bases into a cup at the same time; sprinkle with chocolate powder and you will have a soap which looks like a mocha!

Honey & Dandelion Soap

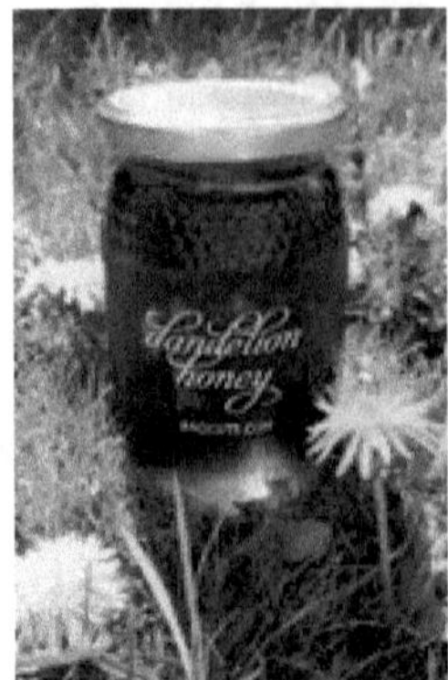

You can use dandelions to make your soap but this may result in bits in your soap! It is better to make a dandelion tea and use this to flavor the soap. The ingredients you will need are are; 10 ounces of dandelion tea and one ounce of honey. These two ingredients need to be added base soap once you have melted it. You should keep the soap simmering to ensure the honey and dandelion tea has mixed completely.

Again, this soap should be set within a few hours; ideally it should be used within three months of its first use.

Cucumber soap

Cucumber is known to clean and refresh any skin, adding it to a soap means you have access to it whenever you need a boost.

To make the soap you will need the pulp of one cucumber. The best way of doing this is to peel and grate it into the smallest pieces possible. Again, you will need to add this to the soap base and warm the entire mixture. It should be set within a few hours.

Soap on a stick

This can be a great way to introduce children to soap and remind everyone of how important it is to wash. Putting soap on a stick may make it appear like a lollipop; you will need to be careful that your children do not try to eat them!

You will need lollipop sticks; clear glycerin, food coloring and fragrance oil. Simply start by cutting the glycerin into blocks and putting them in a bowl before melting them in the microwave. You can then stir in your fragrance, the food coloring and any specific flavor your children may want to wash in. The mixture can then be poured into a mold and a lollipop stick attached. To get the soap to set it is best to put the molds in the freezer for ten minutes.

Conclusion

Making soap is cost effective, fun and will allow you to be extremely creative. There are literally hundreds of recipes, some will use lye whilst others use old soaps or soap base. It can often be good to start with the soap bases and move up to using lye mixtures. This will ensure you are comfortable with all the processes and measuring before tackling the more dangerous approach.

Providing you adopt a cautious approach to lye and always have a bottle of vinegar on standby you will be perfectly safe and capable of using lye. It does give off noxious fumes when first mixed, if possible it is better to mix it outside. However, providing you adopt the right approach you will not have an issue using this product.

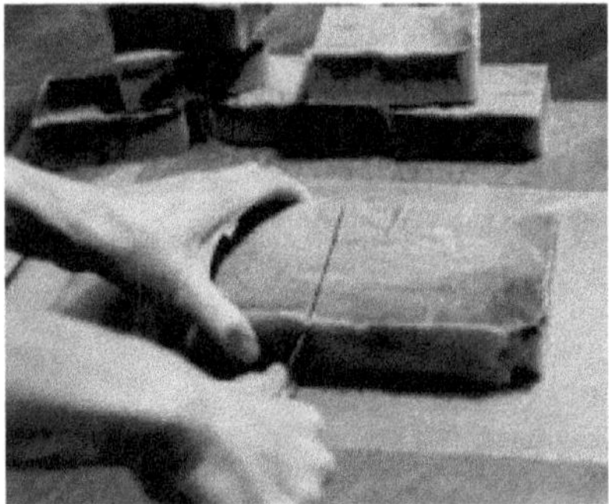

It is also fascinating to note how the scent and even the feel of soap can be completely changed just by increasing or decreasing the quantities of the ingredients. There is no reason why you cannot adjust the quantities or even add extra items to any recipe to make your own variant of soap; at the worst it will not work properly and you can simply start again!

Making your own soap is becoming increasingly popular; this is not just because it is much cheaper than buying luxury soap; there is also a sense of satisfaction and achievement when you make your first batch. In fact, it is so easy to get started in that there is really no excuse for anyone not to have a go!

9 781977 894212